# Pediatric Tricky Topics, Volume 1

Christine M. Houser

# Pediatric Tricky Topics, Volume 1

A Practically Painless Review

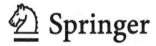 Springer

Christine M. Houser
Department of Emergency Medicine
Erasmus Medical Center
Rotterdam, The Netherlands

ISBN 978-1-4939-1858-4        ISBN 978-1-4939-1859-1 (eBook)
DOI 10.1007/978-1-4939-1859-1
Springer New York Heidelberg Dordrecht London

Library of Congress Control Number: 2014949915

Printed on acid-free paper

Springer is part of Springer Science+Business Media (www.springer.com)

Christine M. Houser

# Pediatric Tricky Topics, Volume 1

A Practically Painless Review

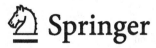 Springer

Christine M. Houser
Department of Emergency Medicine
Erasmus Medical Center
Rotterdam, The Netherlands

ISBN 978-1-4939-1858-4        ISBN 978-1-4939-1859-1 (eBook)
DOI 10.1007/978-1-4939-1859-1
Springer New York Heidelberg Dordrecht London

Library of Congress Control Number: 2014949915

Printed on acid-free paper

Springer is part of Springer Science+Business Media (www.springer.com)

*To my parents, Martin and Cathy, who made this journey possible, to Patrick who travels it with me, and to my wonderful children Tristan, Skyler, Isabelle, Castiel, and Sunderland who have patiently waited during its writing – and are also the most special of all possible reminders of why pediatric medicine is so important.*

# Important Notice

Medical knowledge and the accepted standards of care change frequently. Conflicts are also found regularly in the information provided by various recognized sources in the medical field. Every effort has been made to ensure that the information contained in this publication is as up to date and accurate as possible. However, the parties involved in the publication of this book and its component parts, including the author, the content reviewers, and the publisher, do not guarantee that the information provided is in every case complete, accurate, or representative of the entire body of knowledge for a topic. We recommend that all readers review the current academic medical literature for any decisions regarding patient care.

# Preface

Keeping all of the relevant information at your fingertips in a field as broad as pediatrics is both an important task and quite a lot to manage. Add to that the busy schedule most physicians and physicians-to-be carry of a practice or medical studies, family life, and sundry other personal and professional obligations, and it can be daunting. Whether you would like to keep your knowledge base up to date for your practice, are preparing for the general pediatric board examination or recertification, or are just doing your best to be well prepared for a ward rotation, *Practically Painless Pediatric Tricky Topics, Volume 1* can be an invaluable asset.

This book brings together the information from several major pediatric board review study guides, and more review conferences than any one physician would ever have time to personally attend, for you to review at your own pace. It's important, especially if there isn't a lot of uninterrupted study time available, to find materials that make the study process as efficient and flexible as possible. What makes this book additionally unusual among medical study guides is its design using "bite-sized" chunks of information that can be quickly read and processed. Most information is presented in a question-and-answer format that improves attention and focus, and ultimately learning. Critically important for most in medicine, it also enhances the speed with which the information can be learned.

Because the majority of information is in question-and-answer (Q&A) format, it is also much easier to use the information in a few minutes of downtime at the hospital or office. You don't need to get deeply into the material to understand what you are reading. Each question and answer is brief – not paragraphs long as is often the case in medical review books – which means that the material can be moved through rapidly, keeping the focus on the most critical information.

At the same time, the items have been written to ensure that they contain the necessary information. Very often, information provided in review books raises as many questions as it answers. This interferes with the study process, because the learner either has to look up the additional information (time loss and hassle) or skip the information entirely – which means not really understanding and learning it. This book keeps answers self-contained, meaning that any needed information is provided either directly in the answer or immediately following it – all without lengthy text.

To provide additional study options, questions and answers are arranged in a simple two-column design, making it possible to easily cover one side and quiz yourself, or use the book for quizzing in pairs or study groups.

For a few especially challenging topics, or for the occasional topic that is better presented in a regular text style, a text section has been provided. These sections precede the larger Q&A section for that topic (so, for example, neurology text sections precede the question-and-answer section for neurology). It is important to note that when text sections are present, they are not intended as an overview or introduction to the Q&A section. They are stand-alone topics simply found to be more usefully presented as clearly written and relatively brief text sections.

The materials utilized in *Practically Painless Pediatrics* have been tested by residents and attendings preparing for the general pediatric board examination, or the recertification examination, to ensure that both the approach and content are on target. All content has also been reviewed by attending and specialist pediatricians to ensure its quality and understandability.

If you are using these materials to prepare for an exam, this can be a great opportunity to thoroughly review the many areas involved in pediatric practice, and to consolidate and refresh the knowledge developed through the years so far. *Practically Painless Pediatrics* books are available to cover the breadth of the topics included in the General Pediatric Board Examination.

The formats and style in which materials are presented in *Practically Painless Pediatrics* utilize the knowledge gained about learning and memory processes over many years of research into cognitive processing. All of us involved in the process of creating it sincerely hope that you will find the study process a bit less onerous with this format, and that it becomes – at least at times – an exciting adventure to refresh or build your knowledge.

## Brief Guidance Regarding Use of the Book

Items which appear in **bold** indicate topics known to be frequent board examination content. On occasion, an item's content is known to be very specific to previous board questions. In that case, the item will have "popular exam item" or "item of interest" beneath it.

Some topics cross over between different subjects; for example osteomyelitis is relevant to both the Practically Painless Pediatrics Infectious Disease book and the orthopedic section of this book. In that case, items on the topic will be present in both books, although more extensive coverage of certain aspects will be found in one versus the other. Similarly, various topics overlap between trauma, orthopedics, and environmental medicine. To preserve completeness of coverage, some items for those topics will be found in each of the sections; however, complete repetition of the items in multiple sections would render the chapters unnecessarily long. It is therefore important to review all three sections to ensure a full coverage of the relevant material.

At times, you will encounter a Q&A item that covers the same content as a previous item within the same chapter. These items are worded differently, and often require you to process the information in a somewhat different way, compared to the previous version. This variation in the way questions from particularly challenging or important content areas are asked is not an error or oversight. It is simply a way to easily and automatically practice the information again. These occasionally repeated items are designed to increase the probability that the reader will be able to retrieve the information when it is needed – regardless of how the vignette is presented on the exam, or how the patient presents in a clinical setting.

Occasionally, a brand name for a medication or piece of medical equipment is included in the materials. These are indicated with the trademark symbol (®) and are not meant to indicate an endorsement of, or recommendation to use, that brand name product. Brand names are sometimes included only to make processing of the study items easier, in cases in which the brand name is significantly more recognizable to most physicians than the generic name would be.

The specific word choice used in the text may at times seem informal to the reader, and occasionally a bit irreverent. Please rest assured that no disrespect is intended to anyone or any discipline, in any case. The mnemonics or comments provided are only intended to make the material more memorable. The informal wording is often easier to process than the rather complex or unusual wording many of us in the medical field have become accustomed to. That is why rather straightforward wording is sometimes used, even though it may at first seem unsophisticated.

Similarly, visual space is provided on the page, so that the material is not closely crowded together. This improves the ease of using the material for self- or group quizzing, and minimizes time potentially wasted identifying which answers belong to which questions.

The reader is encouraged to use the extra space surrounding items to make notes or add comments for himself or herself. Further, the Q&A format is particularly well suited to marking difficult or important items for later review & quizzing. If you are utilizing the book for exam preparation, please consider making a system in advance to indicate which items you'd like to return to, which items have already been repeatedly reviewed, and which items do not require further review. This not only makes the study process more efficient & less frustrating, it can also offer a handy way to know which items are most important for last-minute review – frequently a very difficult "triage" task as the examination time approaches.

Finally, consider switching back and forth between topics under review, to improve processing of new items. Trying to learn & remember many information items on similar topics is often more difficult than breaking the information into chunks by periodically switching to a different topic.

Ultimately, the most important aspect of learning the material needed for board and ward examinations is what we as physicians can bring to our patients – and the amazing gift that patients entrust to us in letting us take an active part in their health.

With that focus in mind, the task at hand is not substantially different from what each examination candidate has already done successfully in medical school & in patient care. Keeping that uppermost in our minds, board examination studying should be both a bit less anxiety provoking and a bit more palatable. Seize the opportunity and happy studying to all!

Rotterdam, The Netherlands                                             Christine M. Houser

# About the Author

**Dr. Christine M. Houser** completed her medical degree at the Johns Hopkins University School of Medicine, after spending 4 years in graduate training and research in Cognitive Neuropsychology at George Washington University and the National Institutes of Health. Her Master of Philosophy degree work focused on the processes involved in learning and memory, and during this time she was a four-time recipient of training awards from the National Institutes of Health (NIH). Dr. Houser's dual interests in cognition and medicine led her naturally toward teaching, and "translational cognitive science" – finding ways to apply the many years of cognitive research findings about learning and memory to how physicians and physicians-in-training might more easily learn and recall the vast quantities of information required for medical studies and practice.

# Content Reviewers

Many thanks to Dr. Robert Yetman, Professor and Director of the Residency Program in the Division of Community and General Pediatrics at the University of Texas-Houston Medical School in Houston, Texas, for his tireless assistance in reviewing the manuscript, and coordinating its content review.

## For Orthopedics Topics

Camilo E. Gutiérrez, MD
Assistant Professor of Pediatrics
Boston University School of Medicine
Boston, MA, USA

Mark D. Hormann, MD
Assistant Professor of Pediatrics
University of Texas – Houston Medical School
Houston, TX, USA

## For Trauma, Environmental Medicine, and Toxicology Topics

Rebecca Liggin, MD, FAAP
Associate Professor of Pediatrics and Emergency Medicine
Director of International Medical Education
University of Arkansas School of Medical Sciences
Little Rock, AR, USA

## For General Prevention Topics

Amalia Guardiola, MD
Assistant Professor of Pediatrics
University of Texas – Houston Medical School
Houston, TX, USA

**For Research and Statistics Topics**

Mfon Ekong, MD
Assistant Professor of Pediatrics
University of Texas – Houston Medical School
Houston, TX, USA

**For Rheumatology Topics**

Jonathan S. Hausmann, MD
Fellow in Rheumatology
Harvard Medical School
Children's Hospital Boston
Boston, MA, USA

**For Neurology Topics**

Wendy K. M. Liew, MBChB, MRCPCH
Neuromuscular Fellow
Children's Hospital Boston
Boston, MA, USA

Shih-Ning Liaw, MD
Assistant Professor of Pediatrics
University of Texas – Houston Medical School
Houston, TX, USA

# Contents

# Chapter 1
# General Orthopedics Question and Answer Items

| | |
|---|---|
| Fall on an outstretched hand most commonly results in what two fractures? | 1. Scaphoid<br>2. Colles' fracture (distal radius fracture)<br><br>(Colles' fracture also known as the "dinner fork deformity" – seen mainly in adults) |
| Which type of fracture most commonly injures the radial nerve? | Humeral fracture – *midshaft* |
| What important motor job does the radial nerve do for us? | <u>R</u>adial<br><u>R</u>aises<br>the w<u>R</u>ist |
| **What sensory function does the radial nerve do?** | 1. **<u>Back</u> of the forearm**<br>2. **<u>Back</u> of the hand**<br>3. **<u>Back</u> of first 3 digits (halfway up the fingers)** |
| **Ulnar nerve damage produces what type of problem?** | **Claw hand**<br>(can't abduct fingers) |
| What is the ulnar nerve's main motor job? | Finger abduction<br><br>(also wrist & MCP flexion) |
| **In terms of bone trauma, when is the ulnar nerve most likely to be injured?** | **Posterior elbow dislocation**<br>(it sits in the "ulnar groove" – the funny bone spot!) |
| Which artery is most likely to be damaged in an elbow dislocation? | The brachial artery |

© Springer Science+Business Media New York 2015
C.M. Houser, *Pediatric Tricky Topics, Volume 1*,
DOI 10.1007/978-1-4939-1859-1_1

With any significant dislocation (elbow, knee, ankle) what is the most important step in management?

Reduce the dislocation ASAP

(if this cannot be accomplished immediately – splint it!)

What is the common name for lateral epicondylitis?

Tennis elbow

**What is a nursemaid's elbow?**

**Radial head subluxation**

**How is a nursemaid's elbow usually reduced?**

**Supination + flexion at the elbow**
(gentle pressure on the radial head also helps)

**OR**

**Hyperpronation**

**Should a nursemaid's elbow be X-rayed?**

**No – not needed before or after reduction**

What percentage of children with a nursemaid's elbow will have a reoccurrence?

About 25 %

**Should a nursemaid's elbow be splinted after reduction?**

**No**

What post-reduction management is required for a nursemaid's elbow?

None, except for education on how to prevent them

**What is a "nightstick" fracture?**

**An ulnar fracture**

(as if you were protecting yourself from someone with a nightstick)

Are nightstick fractures displaced, or nondisplaced?

Either

How are nightstick fractures managed?

Displaced – surgically plated into anatomic position to maintain forearm ROM

Nondisplaced – cast

What is Tinel's sign, and what does it indicate?

Tapping on the volar wrist (over the median nerve) produces paresthesia

(indicates carpal tunnel syndrome – *usual treatment rest/NSAIDs/splint*)

What is Phalen's sign?

Sustained pressure on the volar wrist causes paresthesia – "drooping" the hands at the wrists has the same effect

(indicates carpal tunnel syndrome)

In addition to repetitive actions, what are four other risk factors for carpal tunnel syndrome?

Pregnancy
Hypothyroidism
Diabetes
Rheumatoid arthritis

**Which X-ray finding almost invariably indicates an elbow fracture?**

*Posterior* fat pad

What nerve is likely to be damaged by a proximal humerus fracture?

Axillary nerve

How is axillary nerve function tested?

Test deltoid muscle strength

&

Sensation of the overlying skin

Which two shoulder injuries mean that you definitely need to check axillary nerve function?

Proximal humerus fracture

&

*Shoulder dislocation*

Can radial nerve entrapment occur at the wrist?

No – it's not enclosed there

**What is the "Tea Drinker" mnemonic for the functions of the median nerve?**

**The functions needed for drinking a cup of tea:**

**Pincer grasp
(thumb & index finger in the "okay" position)
Biceps
Pronators
Wrist flexors**

What is Guyon's canal?

The space for the ulnar nerve at the wrist

Can the ulnar nerve be entrapped at Guyon's canal?

Yes –
Usually due to external compression

(for example, from bicycle handlebars or a desk surface with computer mouse use)

**Which fracture most often produces a Volkmann's contracture?**

**A supracondylar fracture of the elbow (the humerus at the elbow, specifically)**

What causes Volkmann's contracture?

Inadequate circulation – producing fibrosis and death of forearm soft tissues

*(brachial artery obstruction)*

What causes "swan neck" deformity of a finger?

A tear or avulsion of the extensor tendon for the distal phalanx that goes untreated

*(may result from trauma, rheumatoid arthritis, or other degenerative & inflammatory conditions)*

What is another name for a "swan neck" deformity?

Mallet finger

(because the end hangs down like a mallet)

**If you diagnose a mallet finger, what should you do about it?**

**Splint it from the top (dorsal splint) *in extension* – Ortho follow-up for wiring**

(the tendon and bone need to be together for it to heal properly)

**What is a boxer's fracture?**

**Fracture at the neck of the 5th metacarpal (just proximal to the knuckle)**

**How does a boxer's fracture happen?**

**Axial load landing on a closed fist (e.g., punching a wall)**

How is a boxer's fracture usually treated?

Closed reduction and casting

What is a Bennett's fracture?

A non-comminuted fracture at the base of the thumb (the proximal phalanx is fractured, including the articular surface)

How does a Bennett's fracture happen?

Axial loading on a closed fist (e.g., punching a wall, with too much force going to the thumb)

Which two named fractures refer to fractures at the base of the thumb?

Bennett's and Rolando's fractures

(Rolando's is comminuted & less common)

How are Bennett's and Rolando's fractures managed?

Surgically
(both involve the articular surface of the thumb)

**If a fracture includes the articular surface of a joint, what management is usually required?**

**Operative
(not necessarily immediate, though)**

Which flexor tendon only goes to the middle phalanx?

The flexor digitorum superficialis

Which flexor tendon goes to the end of the finger?

The flexor digitorum profundus
(it's profound – it goes the whole way)

**How is a subungual hematoma treated?**

**Trephination and drainage
(meaning, put a hole through the nail)**

What two tests should be positive with an anterior cruciate ligament tear?

The Lachman and anterior drawer tests

If you have a choice, which test is better for diagnosing anterior cruciate ligament tears – Lachman or anterior drawer?

Lachman

How is the Lachman test performed?

1. Knee is flexed at just 20–30°
   (vs. 90° for anterior drawer)
2. Thigh is stabilized
3. Tibia is pulled forward
*ANY ANTERIOR MOVEMENT IS ABNORMAL*

The anterior drawer test is especially unreliable in what setting?

Acute injury

What type of injury often produces false positives on either the Lachman or the anterior drawer test?

*Posterior* cruciate ligament injury

What is the most common cause of hip pain in children?

Transient synovitis

How do you make a diagnosis of transient synovitis, as a cause for hip pain in a child?

By excluding all of the bad reasons (like fracture, infection, avascular necrosis, or SCFE)

What does SCFE stand for?

Slipped
Capital
Femoral
Epiphysis

Who most commonly develops SCFE?

Obese adolescent boys

Why are pelvic fractures so dangerous?
   (2)

1. The force required to break the pelvis often means that other injuries are present
2. Bleeding is not compressible (so it's hard to control)

Is a double break in the pelvic ring stable or unstable?

Unstable

(there is a strong risk of bleeding and visceral injuries because the separate pieces can move and injure other structures)

**Why are "unstable" joint fractures important to recognize?**

**They require:**
**1. Surgical management**
**2. Total non-weight bearing**

Does patellar tendon damage affect the knee joint?

No

(the patella is a sesamoid bone, so it forms on its own, outside the knee joint)

What function is lost when the quadriceps tendon is ruptured?

Can't extend the knee

(surgical repair is required)

How is a patellar dislocation reduced?

Extend the leg and put gentle medial pressure on the patella
(it usually dislocates laterally, so medial pressure puts it back)

**What is a Baker's cyst?**

**Inflammation of a bursa behind the knee joint**
(several different bursa are present & can cause it)

| | |
|---|---|
| **How does a Baker's cyst present?** | **Painful, swollen popliteal fossa or calf** |
| | **(if it ruptures, the whole calf can swell)** |

**What does SCIWORA stand for?**

**S**pinal
**C**ord
**I**njury
**WithO**ut
**R**adiographic
**A**bnormality

**Which patients are at risk for SCIWORA?**

**Pediatric patients**
**(most often seen in children ≤10 years old)**

**What really happens in SCIWORA?**

**Children's hyperflexible vertebrae can move a long way without being damaged, but the spinal cord cannot**

**(so the X-rays look fine, but the cord is still damaged)**

**What is the prognosis for recovery of function with SCIWORA in a child over 10 years old?**

**Good**

**What is the prognosis for recovery of function with SCIWORA in a child under 10 years old?**

**Poor**

**What is the most important step in the initial management of SCIWORA?**

**IV steroid administration**

Why is SCIWORA usually seen in pediatric patients?

In adults, the force required to damage the spinal cord will usually damage the vertebrae, as well

If a patient suffers a spinal cord injury, but has "sacral sparing," what does that mean for prognosis?

It is good – it indicates that at least part of the cord is intact – 30–50 % recovery

What is "sacral sparing?"

Motor & sensory in the anal/perianal area is intact

(although there are deficits higher up)

| | |
|---|---|
| Is a single break in the pelvic ring dangerous? | Not usually<br><br>(Not likely to cause significant bleeding or additional injury) |
| When is a clavicle fracture worrisome? | If it is near the sternum (middle 1/3)<br><br>• Otherwise no treatment needed |
| Why are certain clavicle fractures worrisome? | Bleeding –<br>Big vessels are close by, and may also be injured |
| **What does the median nerve supply?** | **The palm & adjacent fingers (except for the ulnar part)**<br><br>&<br><br>**Distal half of digits 2, 3, & half of 4, on the back of the hand**<br><br>(wraps around the tips of the fingers, ending its innervation at the PIP joint) |
| **So for which fingers, specifically, does the median nerve provide sensation?** | **Digits 2, 3, and ½ of 4 (thumb also, of course)** |
| **The ulnar nerve provides sensation to which fingers?** | **Fifth finger and medial half of the fourth**<br><br>**(the half of the fourth digit that is closest to the fifth digit)** |
| **Which dermatome does the pinky? Which one does the thumb?** | **Pinky = C8**<br><br>**Thumb = C6**<br><br>(C7 does the area in between) |
| **What is a paronychia, and how is it treated?** | • **An infection of the nail bed (usually near the nail crease)**<br>• **I & D and warm soaks** |
| **Should a patient receive antibiotics after I & D of a paronychia?** | **No – not ordinarily** |
| **Osgood-Schlatter disease – What is it? Who gets it?** | • **Pain over the anterior tibial tuberosity**<br>• **Active adolescent males (mainly)** |

| | |
|---|---|
| **What is osteochondritis dissecans? What does it cause?** | • **A loose body (from the joint) in the knee joint space**<br>• **Pain & locking of the knee joint** |
| What problem can result from prolonged shoulder immobilization? (Prolonged being more than 3 days) | Adhesive capsulitis (frozen shoulder) |
| **What's a greenstick fracture?** | **A pediatric long bone fracture in which only one side of the cortex is disrupted**<br><br>(like when you bend a "green stick," and the bark pops open on just one side) |
| **How is radial nerve motor function tested?** | **Radial Raises the wRist (and extends the fingers – makes sense – it runs along the back of the forearm)** |
| **How do you test ulnar nerve motor function?** | **Finger abduction/ adduction**<br><br>(technically, you're testing the strength of the "lumbricals" in the hand) |
| **What is the easiest way to test median nerve function?** | **Make the "OK" sign**<br><br>(the patient, not you) |
| What are six significant complications of fractures?<br><br>(think vascular complications, infectious complications, bone problems, sudden death problem) | 1. Compartment syndrome<br>2. Fat emboli<br>3. Nonunion or malunion<br>4. Arthritis<br>5. Avascular necrosis<br>6. Osteomyelitis |
| **What is compartment syndrome?** | **Too much pressure in a closed space cuts off the arterial supply to that area – soft tissues die** |
| **What is a Volkmann's contracture?** | **When compartment syndrome kills off the soft tissues in the forearm (most common after supracondylar fracture)** |

**What are the "5 Ps" that indicate your patient might have compartment syndrome?**

1. **Pain (earliest finding – more pain than expected)**
2. **Pallor**
3. **Paresthesia**
4. **Paralysis**
5. **Pulselessness (late finding)**

What are the two main complications of a coccygeal fracture?

1. Coccydynia (chronic pain)
2. Rectal injury (from the sharp bone fragment)

How is a coccygeal fracture diagnosed?

Rectal exam

(feel for the fragment)

What is de Quervain's tenosynovitis?

A painful overuse syndrome of the radial flexor tendons

How is de Quervain's treated?

Rest
Splint
NSAIDs

What is "Finkelstein's test?"

1. Make a fist
2. Bend the wrist toward the ulnar side
3. PAIN!!!

(Ulnar deviation of the wrist, with the hand in a fist, produces pain)

What diagnosis does it suggest?

De Quervain's tenosynovitis

**What type of shoulder dislocation is most common?**

**Anterior dislocation**

**What is the most common complication of a shoulder dislocation?**

**Axillary nerve damage**

How do you test for axillary nerve damage?

Sensation over the deltoid

OR

Arm abduction

What medical condition is most likely to cause a posterior shoulder dislocation?

A seizure

| | |
|---|---|
| **Which nerve is most likely to be damaged in mid-shaft humeral fractures?** | **The radial nerve** <br><br> **(it sits in the "spiral groove" of the humerus)** |
| **What happens if the radial nerve is damaged, in terms of motor function?** | **Wrist drop** |
| **How can you most easily test radial nerve function?** | **1. Motor – Wrist extension** <br> **2. Sensation – First web space** |
| In addition to seizure, in what other situations might you see posterior shoulder dislocations? <br>     (3) | 1. Fall from a height (or other big impact) <br> 2. Lightning strike <br> 3. High-voltage injury |
| What do Kanavel's signs refer to? | Signs of flexor tenosynovitis |
| What are the signs? <br>     (4) | 1. *Fusiform* (sausage-like) finger swelling <br> 2. Pain with *palpation* of the tendon sheath <br> 3. Severe pain with finger *extension* (passive extension) <br> 4. Patient holds finger in *slightly flexed* position |
| How is flexor tenosynovitis treated? | Surgical I & D of the sheath |
| What usually gets a flexor tenosynovitis infection started? | Puncture wound to the volar hand or finger |
| What is anterior cord syndrome? <br><br> How does it happen? | • Motor paralysis distal to lesion, with loss of pain and temperature sensation <br> • Hypotension/vascular accidents or hyperflexion at the neck |
| **What is the biggest worry about knee dislocation?** | • **Injury to the popliteal artery** |
| **Why?** | • **It's tethered around the knee** |
| **What is the second biggest worry?** | **Damage to the (deep) peroneal nerve – causes "foot drop"** |
| **What is the initial management of a scaphoid fracture?** | **Splinting to above the elbow & immobilize thumb** |

| | |
|---|---|
| **What is the most common complication of a scaphoid fracture?** | **Avascular necrosis, leading to arthritis** |
| **Of the carpal bones, which one is fractured most often?** | **The scaphoid** |
| **What physical finding should make you automatically treat for a scaphoid fracture?** | **Pain in the "snuff box" area with palpation** *(X-rays are often negative!)* |
| **If a patient injured the wrist/ hand area, and now has tenderness in the snuff box area, but no other findings on physical or X-ray, what should you do?** | **Splint and refer for ortho follow-up** (It's a scaphoid fracture until proven otherwise!) |
| **What does a positive Ortolani sign indicate?** | **Developmental dysplasia of the hip (aka hip dysplasia,** *formerly known as "congenital hip dislocation")* |
| Is developmental dysplasia of the hip more common in girls or boys? | Females (80 %) |
| What causes developmental dysplasia of the hip? | Excessive joint laxity |
| How do we check for developmental dysplasia of the hip (DDH)? | Ortolani & Barlow maneuvers |
| What are three common risk factors for DDH? | 1. Female<br>2. Breech birth<br>3. Dysplasia in the other hip (20 % bilateral) |
| Is there an inherited component to DDH? | Yes –<br>10× increased chance of DDH if a parent also had DDH |
| How is developmental dysplasia of the hip treated in very young infants? | Pavlik harness brace if caught earlier than 8 weeks of age |

| | |
|---|---|
| Which racial backgrounds have an unusually high likelihood of DDH? | Native Americans<br><br>&<br><br>Laplanders(!)<br>(Lapland is an northern area of Finland) |
| Children from which two racial backgrounds have a very low likelihood of DDH? | Chinese<br><br>&<br><br>African American<br>(or other black populations) |
| For children older than 8 weeks, how do we treat DDH? | Traction and spica cast, and occasionally surgery |
| What sign indicates a positive result for the Barlow & Ortolani maneuvers? | A "clunk" |
| How does the Barlow test differ from the Ortolani test? | Barlow is the adduction of flexed hip and knee, Ortolani is abduction of flexed leg |
| How is the hip positioned in early treatment of DDH? | To maintain hip flexion and abduction |
| Too much abduction in the treatment of DDH may lead to what complication? | Femoral head necrosis<br>(due to circumflex artery damage) |
| When treating developmental dysplasia of the hip with a Pavlik harness, too much flexion can lead to what complication? | Nerve palsy |
| Are infants from cultures that use (tight) swaddling at increased risk for DDH? | Yes |
| What does the Allis test tell you? | Whether one femur is "shorter" than the other, indicating unilateral congenital dislocation |
| How is the Allis test performed? | With the patient supine and knees flexed, compare the heights of the two patellas |

| | |
|---|---|
| What is the optimal age to treat developmental dysplasia of the hip? | Before 8 weeks |
| When is surgical correction of DDH required? | If the child is more than 1 year old, or already walking |
| Which tendons are usually released in the treatment of children with clubfoot? | The Achilles, and sometimes the hallucis tendons |
| Which foot abnormality is closely associated with spinal abnormalities? | "Rocker bottom" foot (congenital vertical talus) |
| What is pes calcaneovalgus? | A flexed, outward-oriented foot at birth ("pes" means foot) |
| How is pes calcaneovalgus treated? | Stretching exercises for approximately 3 months |
| What causes pes calcaneovalgus to develop? | Interuterine malpositioning of the foot |
| What is metatarsus varus? | Inward angulation of the metatarsals |
| What is the treatment of metatarsus varus in the older child? | Nothing if asymptomatic – surgical osteotomy needed after age 4 |
| If metatarsus varus is diagnosed before age 4 months, how can it be treated? | Casting, followed by straight shoes until age 2 years |
| What is metatarsus primus varus? | Inward angulation of the *first metatarsal only* |
| Why is treating metatarsus primus varus more important than treating a total metatarsus varus deformity? | The great toe is pushed in a valgus direction by shoes, leading to bunion formation, when only the first metatarsal is affected |
| Should adolescents be referred to surgery for correction of bunions (deformity of the metatarso-phalangeal joint)? | Defer if possible – high recurrence rate |
| What is pes planovalgus? | Flatfoot |

| | |
|---|---|
| What is the problem with having pes planovalgus? | It can cause significant "overpronation" |
| Are corrective shoes required if a pes planovalgus foot has full range of motion? | No |
| What is the treatment for pronation in pes planovalgus? | Orthotics |
| If a pes planovalgus foot does not have full range of motion, what should you suspect? | Other ortho problems such as heel cords, or rocker bottom foot |
| What congenital ortho condition should you suspect if an 8–10-year-old complains of foot pain and stiffness? | Tarsal coalition – tarsals don't segment correctly, and instead ossify together |
| How is tarsal coalition treated? | Surgically |
| **What is Gower's sign?** | **The inability to rise from sitting without using arms, due to weakness of the leg muscles**<br><br>**(photo items usually show a child attempting to rise from the floor, with or without showing use of the arms to help)** |
| What foot deformity is associated with Friedrich's ataxia? | Pes cavus |
| What is the alternate name for spina bifida cystica, which is associated with club foot? | Myelomeningocele |
| What is amyotonia congenita? | Congenital generalized lack of muscle tone & poor muscle bulk |
| What is the inheritance pattern of amyotonia congenita? | There are many underlying disorders – can be dominant, recessive, or X-linked |
| What is the prognosis for amyotonia congenita? | Variable, but usually poor – supportive care only |

| | |
|---|---|
| Has improved prenatal care and fetal monitoring changed the incidence of cerebral palsy? | No |
| Mental retardation is most often associated with which type of cerebral palsy? | Spastic quadriplegia |
| It is unlikely that a child with cerebral palsy will be able to walk, if he/she has not already started walking by what age? | Seven years |
| For young children with cerebral palsy, presence of which reflexes improves the likelihood of walking? | "Parachute" and "stepping" reflexes |
| What is the parachute reflex? | Lifelong reflex that makes our arms fly out when we feel like we're falling |
| What is the stepping reflex? | Before infants can weight bear, they will still "try" to push and step with their legs if supported |
| At what age can you make the diagnosis of cerebral palsy (and also have some idea of prognosis)? | Age 2 |
| Are the bones and joints of cerebral palsy patients abnormal from birth? | Generally, no. (Bone and joint changes happen with growth and spastic muscles) |
| What is one of the most important goals of physical therapy for wheelchair-bound cerebral palsy patients? | A level pelvis allowing a normal sitting position reduces morbidity and increases comfort |
| What are the primary contributing factors to the development of arthrogryposis multiplex congenita? | Aplasia and hypoplasia of multiple muscle groups (with congenital joint contractures) |
| What is the appropriate treatment for children who walk with their toes turned too far in or out? | If it persists for greater than 6 months, corrective night braces can be used |

| | |
|---|---|
| What is normal leg position, in terms of rotation, for most infants? | Internal tibial torsion |
| What are the three most common causes of a limp in a child aged 5–10 years? | Legg-Calve-Perthes disease Transient synovitis Osgood-Schlatter disease |
| What is the typical gait of the newly walking child? | Wide based, with external rotation |
| What simple intervention can assist the correction of "out-toed" walking in the older toddler? | Placing the child to sleep in the "frog-leg" position (Just curious, but do they stay like that voluntarily??) |
| Does the "W" sitting position (medial knee and foot down, toes pointed laterally) help or hinder bone and gait development? | It hinders it by putting stress on the femurs, and making "in-toeing" worse |
| Is cross-legged sitting ("Indian style") good for bone and gait development? | Yes |
| What is the common name for genu varum? (genu = knee) | Bow legs |
| Is genu varum ever normal in children? | Yes – usually resolves between 18 and 36 months |
| What is the common name for genu valgum? | Knock knees |
| Is genu valgum ever normal in children? | Yes – Common in 3–6 year olds (resolves spontaneously) |
| What is the differential diagnosis of severe or persistent genu valgus or varus? | Rickets Dwarfism Renal osteodystrophy (in the presence of renal disease, of course) |
| What is the recommended management of a child with a lower extremity length discrepancy of less than 3 cm? | Observation |

| | |
|---|---|
| What is the recommended management of a child with a lower extremity length discrepancy of 3–6 cm? | Limb shortening |
| What is the recommended management of a child with a lower extremity length discrepancy of greater than 6 cm? | Limb lengthening |
| What is the differential diagnosis of joint effusion in a child? (5 possibilities) | 1. Trauma<br>2. Septic joint<br>3. Hemophilia (or other bleeding disorder)<br>4. Rheumatological disease<br>5. Inflammator infusion (transient synovitis) |
| **What is the underlying pathology in Legg-Calve-Perthes disease?** | **Avascular necrosis of the femoral head in a growing child** |
| Legg-Calve-Perthes is sometimes written three different ways. What are they? | Legg-Calve-Perthes<br>Perthes disease<br>Calve-Perthes<br><br>*They are all the same – don't worry about it* |
| What is the prognosis of Legg-Calve-Perthes disease in a child less than 6 years old? | Usually good (without treatment) |
| What is the prognosis of Perthes disease in a child older than 10? | Usually poor |
| **In addition to limping, children with Perthes disease often complain of pain at what two sites?** | **Hip &<br>Knee** |
| In Calve-Perthes disease, hip motion is most limited in what direction? | Extension (abduction can also be affected) |
| What is the usual treatment for Legg-Calve-Perthes disease when treatment is needed? | A brace – abduction with internal rotation position |

| | |
|---|---|
| What is the purpose of "containment bracing" in the treatment of Legg-Perthes disease? | To mold the femoral head as it re-ossifies |
| Is hip range of motion limited in transient synovitis? | Sometimes |
| What laboratory test results reinforce a diagnosis of transient synovitis? | CBC and ESR should both be in the normal range |
| What joint does Osgood-Schlatter disease affect? | The knee |
| What is Osgood-Schlatter disease? | Inflammation of the tibial tubercle |
| What patient group most often develops Osgood-Schlatter disease? | Adolescent boys involved in sports |
| How is Osgood-Schlatter disease usually treated? | Rest, NSAIDs, and a knee brace |
| How is Osgood-Schlatter disease treated on the rare occasions when standard management is not effective? | Surgical excision of the inflamed point of the ossicle |
| What must always be in the differential diagnosis of knee pain? | Hip problem |
| In slipped capital femoral epiphysis (SCFE), is the slippage acute or gradual? | Trick question, all are possible – Can be acute, gradual, or sometimes acute on gradual |
| SCFE patients won't want to move their leg in which direction, especially? | Internal rotation |
| What are the consequences of congenitally missing clavicles? | None<br><br>(Houdini used this to his advantage) |
| What is Sprengel's deformity? | Abnormal location of the scapula (due to a problem with embryological migration) |

| | |
|---|---|
| How does Sprengel's deformity look? | Like one scapula is missing |
| *Is* the scapula missing in Sprengel's deformity? | No, it is abnormally high and recessed |
| What radiological study is required to clear a Down syndrome patient for sports participation? | A cervical spine series to rule out atlanto-axial instability |
| How is torticollis usually treated in children? | Stretching exercises |
| What characteristics are seen in a patient with Klippel-Feil syndrome? | Webbed neck, low hairline in back, and *congenital failure of cervical spine segmentation* |
| At what age should children be screened for idiopathic scoliosis? | Age 10 |
| What degree of curvature in scoliosis requires treatment with a brace? | Greater than 25° |
| Does pain occur in scoliosis? | No, consider a tumor if present |
| Why is scoliosis not treated after the skeleton is mature? | It is not effective<br>+<br>scoliosis doesn't worsen after skeletal maturity |
| What are the measurements used to evaluate scoliosis called? | Cobb measurements |
| What type of scoliosis is associated with neurological problems? | Left thoracic |
| At what degree of curvature must surgical correction of scoliosis be performed for medical versus cosmetic reasons? | Greater than 40° |
| Can scoliosis be present congenitally? | Yes, there can be rib or spinal abnormalities, or infantile thoracotomy can produce it |

"Growing pains" at night relieved by aspirin/NSAIDS are suggestive of what diagnosis?

Osteoid osteoma

Do children get vertebral disc herniations?

Yes, they sometimes present as a painful scoliosis

Where do children with a herniated disk complain of pain?

In the leg, as opposed to the back

Bone scans often help with the diagnosis of what three problems?

Stress fractures
Osteomyelitis
Discitis

What is the preferred study for diagnosing disc herniation?

MRI

What physical exam sign is likely to be positive in a patient with a herniated disc?

Straight leg raise or crossed straight leg raise
(when you raise the unaffected leg, the patient feels pain on the *other side*)

Is surgery usually indicated in children with disc herniation?

No – high failure rate

In addition to disc herniation, MRI is especially useful for diagnosing what other sort of important spinal growths?

Intraspinal tumors

What is diastematomyelia?

A long, cartilaginous cleft in the spinal cord

Occult spinal dysraphisms, including diastematomyelia, present with what signs and symptoms?

Urinary incontinence
Leg weakness
Gait problems, and
Foot deformity

What is the most common cause of low back pain in adolescents?

Poor posture

Can poor posture be corrected?

Yes – physical therapy can be quite helpful

What is Scheuermann's kyphosis?

A fixed, structural kyphosis of the thoracic spine, affecting three or more vertebrae

| | |
|---|---|
| Which sex is more likely to develop Scheuermann's kyphosis? | Males |
| Can discitis be diagnosed based on physical exam and radiology alone? | No – needle biopsy and culture are required |
| What disorder must be ruled out in any child with birth fractures? | Osteogenesis imperfecta must be considered (although many normal infants have birth fractures) |
| How are birth-related clavicle fractures treated? | They are not treated – heal within 10 days |
| How are birth-related femur fractures treated? | Traction for 3 weeks |
| What diagnoses should be considered in a child with low back and poorly localized extremity pain, not associated with activity? | Spondyloarthropathies, such as ankylosing, spondylitis OR Malignancy (e.g., leukemia) |
| What sex and HLA group are associated with the spondyloarthropathies? | Male sex & HLA-B27 positive |
| In the reduction of a long bone fracture, which directional alignment is most important? | Rotational alignment |
| What factor determines the amount of displacement and angulation that can remain after a fracture reduction? | The younger a patient is, the more angulation and displacement are allowed |
| Which Salter-Harris fracture type is a slipped capital femoral epiphysis? | Type I |
| Do long bone fractures in children require anatomic reduction? | Only in the rotational plane |
| Why is anatomic reduction not critical in children? | Because extensive remodeling will occur, correcting most misalignment |

| | |
|---|---|
| Which Salter-Harris-type fractures require anatomic reduction? | Types III and IV |
| Which humeral fracture requires close monitoring and management? | Supracondylar fractures—malunion and Volkmann's contracture can occur |
| What is a common sequelae of supracondylar fracture? | Elbow stiffness |
| Are weight-bearing exercises, or physical therapy, indicated to improve ROM in supracondylar fractures? | No—ROM improves with time |
| What causes "gunstock deformity" of the arm?<br><br>(looks like a hump in the arm) | Malunion and/or rotary misalignment after a supracondylar fracture |
| How is the "gunstock deformity" corrected? | Surgically |
| Should gunstock deformity be corrected routinely? | No – it is often a cosmetic issue only |
| At what age should children's fractures be treated the same as adult fractures? | Age 14 |
| What technique is often used to improve the angulation of greenstick fractures? | Completing the fracture |
| If the positioning of a fracture is described as "bayonet" fracture alignment, what does that mean? | One end of the fracture overrides the other<br><br>(looks like an old-fashioned bayonet design) |
| Is "overriding" in a femur fracture acceptable? | Yes – the leg can lengthen at the epiphysis to compensate<br>(bizarre!) |
| What form of traction is commonly used in femur fractures of very small children? | Skin traction |

Why can traction in pediatric fractures result in a lengthened extremity?

The traction stimulates growth at the epiphysis

Why is ORIF (open reduction/ internal fixation) generally not used to treat femur fractures in children?

There is a high rate of osteomyelitis and nonunion

How are tibial shaft fractures treated in children?

With closed reduction and casting

How are metatarsal and toe fractures usually treated?

With a walking boot (a rigid flat-soled shoe) for several weeks

Fractures involving which bone surface always require surgical correction?

The articular (joint) surface

Which tarsal bone is fractured most often?

The calcaneus

What is the most common mechanism for a calcaneus fracture?

A fall from a height

What other injury is associated with calcaneal fractures?

L2–L5 fractures

(finding a calcaneal fracture should always make you evaluate the lumbar spine)

**What are four signs of meniscal injury?**

**Catching**
**Locking**
**"Giving way"**
**Pain while climbing stairs**

**What factor is the main determinant of whether hand fractures require surgical pinning?**

**Finger alignment and hand grip must be preserved**

**What is a felon?**
**(in medicine, that is)**

**An infection in the pulp space of the finger tip**

**How are felons treated?**

**With I & D and antibiotics**

**What does a posterior fad pad indicate on an elbow radiograph?**

**The presence of a radial head fracture** (can sometimes be a supracondylar fracture, also)

**What is the common name for a torus fracture?**

**Buckle fracture**

What is a Lisfranc dislocation?

A traumatic dislocation between the tarsals and the metatarsals, so they no longer line up

Which part of the spine is affected by Chance fractures?

The lumbar spine (vertebral body disruption)

What mechanism most often causes Chance fractures?

A motor vehicle accident when wearing a lap belt without a shoulder belt

Are Chance fractures stable or unstable?

Unstable – risk of spinal cord injury

What is a third-degree ankle sprain?

Complete rupture of ankle ligaments

Which ligament is most commonly injured in ankle sprains?

The anterior talofibular

(talofibular is easy to remember – you know that most people injure the *outer* ankle, where the talus connects to the fibula)

What are the signs of Achilles tendon rupture?
(3)

1.  Bruising at the posterior ankle/foot
2.  Soft concave area at the back of the ankle
3.  Positive Thompson's test
(no plantar flexion when the calf is squeezed)

How is an Achilles tendon rupture treated?

Splinting in plantar flexion, then usually surgical repair

**What are two simple techniques to evaluate median nerve function?**

**Make an "OK" sign with the hand**
&
**Flex the index and middle fingers**

What is a Jeffersonian, or burst fracture?

The bony ring of the C1 vertebra bursts outward in multiple pieces

How does a Jeffersonian fracture usually occur?

From an axial load on the head, such as an auto passenger hitting the roof (or a diving injury)

Which vertebrae most commonly develop burst fractures?

The cervical vertebrae

Are burst fractures stable or unstable?

Unstable – surgical repair

What is the typical appearance of a patient with a posterior hip dislocation?

The lower extremity is flexed and internally rotated

(sometimes called "embarrassed swimmer's" position)

What is the typical mechanism for a posterior hip dislocation?

MVC while passenger traveling with foot on the dashboard

(can sometimes happen with knee impact on dashboard)

**What is the most common complication of a hip fracture?**

**Avascular necrosis**

What is the most common type of hip fracture?

An intertrochanteric fracture

(literally goes between the greater and lesser trochanter of the hip – makes sense, because that's the part of the hip that sticks out)

**What is the most common finding in rotator cuff injuries?**

**Pain and limited ROM with abduction and external rotation**

**What is the most commonly injured knee ligament in kids?**

**Medial collateral**

**Why are femur fractures dangerous?**

**Blood loss (one liter easily)**

**&**

**Fat emboli**

**What is the most common pathogen in septic arthritis?**

**Staph aureus**

**What is the most common "special" pathogen causing septic arthritis in sickle cell patients?**

**Salmonella**

| | |
|---|---|
| **What does the "Boutonniere" finger deformity look like?** | **PIP is flexed, DIP is extended** |
| **What causes the Boutonniere deformity?** | **Rupture or dislocation of the central extensor tendon from its attachment on the middle phalanx** |
| What two methods are used to manage carpal tunnel syndrome? | Rest/splinting/NSAIDs<br><br>Or<br><br>Surgical release of the median nerve in the carpal tunnel |
| When is surgical correction required for metacarpal fractures? | When rotation of the fractured metacarpal interferes with grip<br><br>(>5° of rotation is a problem) |
| **Why is rotation so important in metacarpal fractures?** | **Because if the metacarpal is rotated too far, the finger alignment suffers, and grip strength is lost**<br><br>**(You can't hold a beer can anymore!)** |
| **If you are a metacarpal, how much rotation is too much, in general terms?** | **As you might guess, the closer you are to the thumb, the straighter you must be!** |
| How much angulation is permitted in the various metacarpal fractures to ensure function? | 5th—45°<br>4th—35°<br>3rd—15°<br>2nd—15°<br><br>(the closer it is to the thumb, the less rotation is okay) |
| **Is any treatment required after reduction of a patellar dislocation?** | **No**<br>**(a knee immobilizer is usually provided for stability)** |
| What is the danger of a medial clavicle fracture? | Injury to the great vessels nearby |
| **How is flexor tenosynovitis different from tendonitis?** | **Tenosynovitis is an infection (& it's an emergency),**<br><br>**tendonitis is inflammatory** |

| | |
|---|---|
| **How is flexor tenosynovitis treated?** | **Surgical I & D by an ortho or hand specialist** |
| **What is the main complication of open fractures?** | **Infection** |
| How is the initial management of an open fracture different from closed? | Antibiotics, tetanus prophylaxis, and lavage are required |
| What is a Charcot joint? | Poorly defined bony outlines (usually in the ankle), caused by multiple fractures/trauma/ arthritis |
| What underlying problem leads to Charcot joint? | Lack of sensation and proprioception |
| Who typically develops Charcot joints? | Diabetics, and other patients with peripheral neuropathies |
| **How many categories are in the original Salter-Harris fracture classification system?** | **Five** |
| **Which Salter fracture has the worse prognosis?** | **Type 5 – Possibility of no further growth! – plate compressed onto metaphysis** |
| **Which Salter fracture is most common, and what does it look like?** | • **Type 2**<br>• **Goes through the plate & *up* into the metaphysis** |
| **Which Salter-Harris fractures go down, through the epiphysis?** | **Types 3 and 4** |
| **How is a Salter 3 different from a Salter 4?** | • **Salter 4 goes *up & down***<br>• **Salter 3 goes through the plate, then *down only*** |
| **Which two Salter-Harris fractures are often "invisible" on X-ray?** | **Types 1 and 5**<br><br>**(Type 1 is slipped or apart)**<br><br>**(Type 5 is compressed)** |

| | |
|---|---|
| **How could you describe the Salter-Harris fractures in order, using one word each?** | **Apart (out)**<br>**Up**<br>**Down**<br>**Through (both)**<br>**In**<br><br>**(Kind of sounds like a workout routine – some students have found that an arm routine helps them to remember which is which!)** |
| **Foot puncture wounds and IV drug abuse habits put you at risk for what unusual type of osteomyelitis (organism)?** | **Pseudomonas** |
| **When "tapping" a knee or bursa, what is the main concern?** | **Introduction of infection** |
| **How is bursitis usually treated?** | **Rest and NSAIDs** |
| **What is pseudosubluxation of the C-spine in pediatrics?** | **A 2–3 mm misalignment of the anterior cervical line**<br><br>*(normal variant in kids less than 8 years old – that's why it's "pseudosubluxation")* |
| What is the anatomically based name for "Blount disease?" | Idiopathic tibia vara |
| Which kids tend to develop Blount disease? | Obese kids<br>(can be any age group – most severe when it starts early) |
| How can you remember what happens in Blount disease? | Think of the weight of the child making the legs "bow out" at the knee |
| What happens to make the legs bow out in Blount disease? | Overgrowth of one side of the tibia at the joint |
| Is Blount disease common? | No |
| How is Blount disease treated? | Usually with bracing – severe cases can be operative |

| | |
|---|---|
| What is a plastic deformity fracture? | No visible fracture BUT Bone is bent beyond its normal limits (there are microfractures not seen on X-ray) |
| Which children are most likely to have a plastic deformity fracture? | Very young children with forearm injuries |
| How are plastic deformity fractures treated? | Closed reduction usually under general anesthesia if it is severe enough to cause cosmetic or functional issues |
| Can plastic deformity fractures be observed & allowed to remodel? | It depends – Remodeling is most successful in children <6 years old, with not very severe deformity |
| What is a Monteggia fracture? | The proximal 1/3 of the ulna fractures, while the radial head dislocates *(ouch!)* |

*Mnemonic:*
*To make an "M" with your arms, fold your hands together in the middle, bending your wrists, then bend your elbow joints a bit. You need to use your elbows & your wrists – Monteggia therefore involves both the wrist (radial head dislocation) and the elbow area (proximal ulnar fracture)*

| | |
|---|---|
| What is a Galeazzi fracture? | The distal 1/3 of the radius fractures, with dislocation of the radial-ulnar joint |

*(Note: This one is generally all distal. The Monteggia involves the area near the elbow.)*

| | |
|---|---|
| What is the order in which the elbow ossification centers mature? | C – capitellum (1 year) R – radial head (3 years) I – inner condyle (5 years) T – trochlea (7 years) O – olecranon (9 years) E – external condyle (11 years) |
| What is a "toddler's fracture?" | A distal tibia fracture when the child is new to walking (about 9 months to 3 years) |

What is the classic mechanism for a toddler's fracture?

A planted foot with rotation

When is a femoral fracture very worrying for child abuse?

If the child is non-ambulatory

Which four fractures are pathognomonic for child abuse?

- Posterior rib fractures
- Spiral fractures in the non-ambulatory
- Metaphyseal (bucket handle) fractures
- Sternal fractures

How is the pattern of C-spine fracture different in young children, compared to adolescents or adults?

High cervical spine fractures are more common (C3 & above)

(older adolescents & adults most typically fracture C6-T1)

Why do younger children have this pattern of C-spine fractures?
   (3 reasons)

Bigger head compared to body

Higher fulcrum for the force

Smaller & weaker neck musculature

What radiological marker is helpful for identifying pseudosubluxation in the C-spine, and how do you use it?

The posterior line (of Swischuk) – Draw a line between the posterior arches of C1 & C3

C2's *anterior* aspect of its posterior arch should be within 2 mm of the line, if it is *pseudo*subluxation

What are the most common sites for osteosarcoma to develop in children?

Distal femur & proximal tibia (around the knee) – 60 %

Proximal femur – 15 %

Proximal humerus – 10 %

What is the usual imaging modality for triplanar ankle fractures?

CT is needed to determine precise arrangement of the fracture

(Do plain films first)

What is "triplanar" about a triplanar ankle fracture?

Coronal, sagittal, & transverse planes of injury are present –

In general:
Metaphysis – coronal fracture
Growth plate – transverse fracture
Epiphysis – sagittal fracture

Why is this injury a uniquely pediatric injury?

It occurs due to asymmetric (uneven) closure of the tibial growth plate during a period of about 18 months

What are Salter-Harris fractures types VI & IX (6 & 9)?

VI – Injury to the perichondral structures (may still affect growth)

IX – Injury to the periosteum, which can affect (membranous) growth

If a child sustains a fracture, and only the epiphyseal plate is damaged, what is the name of that fracture?

Salter-Harris type VII (7)

If the metaphysis only is injured, but in an area that might affect growth, what Salter-Harris name is now given to that fracture?

Salter-Harris type VIII (8)

# Chapter 2
# General Trauma Question and Answer Items

**What are the ABCDEs of trauma resuscitation?**

**A airway intact?**
**B breathing okay?**
**C circulation okay? (& C-spine?)**
**D disability (anything not working?)**
**E exposure (seeing all of the patient)**

**What is the best radiology study for the initial evaluation of possible head injury?**

**Noncontrast head CT**
**(US can only be used in very young infants with open fontanelles & is not recommended for head trauma evaluation)**

**When should you obtain an *emergent* MRI?**

**For possible spinal cord compression**
**(if MRI is available – the images are much better than CT images)**

**What X-rays should be ordered for every major trauma patient?**

**C-spine**
**Chest**
**Pelvis X-ray or CT abdomen/pelvis**

(others as needed, depending on injuries)

In general, what is the correct management for a patient with penetrating abdominal trauma?

Exploratory laparotomy

How do you treat an *open* pneumothorax?
  (2 techniques)

- Use an occlusive dressing to cover three sides of the wound (air gets out, but not into the chest)
- Intubation and positive pressure ventilation may also be needed

© Springer Science+Business Media New York 2015
C.M. Houser, *Pediatric Tricky Topics, Volume 1*,
DOI 10.1007/978-1-4939-1859-1_2

What is the other name for an open pneumothorax?

A sucking chest wound

(the diameter of the opening determines how much sucking it will do – bigger is worse)

**What is the correct treatment for an unstable patient thought to have cardiac tamponade?**

**Pericardiocentesis**

Can penetrating trauma cause cardiac tamponade?

Yes – usually left chest trauma

**What are the five physical findings you should expect with cardiac tamponade?**
*(The first three are known as "Beck's triad.")*

1. **Hypotension**
2. **Distended neck veins**
3. **Muffled heart sounds**
4. **Pulsus paradoxus**
5. *Clear lung sounds*

How do you treat massive hemothorax?

- Chest tube and volume support
- If the bleeding does not stop shortly after insertion of the chest tube, clamp it and get the patient to the OR

**What is the most common cause of a fever in the first 24-h post-op?**

**Atelectasis**

What is a flail chest?

An injury that produces a segment of the chest wall that moves independently from the rest of the chest wall (due to rib fractures)

How do you get a flail chest?

You break multiple, adjacent ribs in *at least two places*
(This allows that segment of chest to "float free" from the rest of the ribs)

Why is flail chest a bad thing?

It causes inadequate respiration due to –
1. Pain
2. Pulmonary contusion
3. Probable shunting due to paradoxical motion
(when the patient tries to breathe in, that part of the chest wall goes in rather than expanding out with the rest)

| | |
|---|---|
| How do you treat flail chest? | 1. Pain meds<br>2. Try to prevent paradoxical motion (lie the patient on the injury,  or sand bag the area)<br>3. Intubation<br>4. Positive pressure ventilation is often necessary |
| What is the most common cause of death that immediately follows a motor vehicle collision? | Head injury |
| What is the most common cause of death that immediately follows a fall from a significant height? | Head injury |
| What puts a patient at risk for aortic rupture? | Rapid deceleration<br><br>(the aorta is "tethered" at the ligamentum arteriosum, and the rapid rotation can damage it) |
| What typically causes diaphragmatic rupture? | Blunt trauma |
| Which side of the diaphragm usually ruptures? | Left side |
| **What is the best thing to do with an avulsed (permanent) tooth?** | **Replace it in the socket ASAP** |
| **Is it alright to clean an avulsed tooth, if it has gotten dirty?** | **Gentle saline wash is alright, if necessary**<br><br>**(but never scrub a tooth!!!)** |
| **What is the best thing to do with an avulsed permanent tooth if the patient cannot keep it in the socket (due to patient age, associated fracture, etc.)** | **1. Put it in "Hanks' solution"**<br>**2. Put it in milk if you don't have the special solution** |
| **What is the best thing to do with an avulsed deciduous tooth?** | **Nothing –**<br>**See a dentist for follow-up** |

**What should you do for a
choking victim who is still
breathing?**

**Observe only.
They will usually clear the object on
their own.**

**What should you do for a
choking victim who stops
breathing?**

- **Heimlich if they stop breathing**
- **Abdominal thrust if they pass out**
- **Back blows are for very young
  children**

**What are the signs of a tension
pneumothorax?
(3)**

**Tracheal deviation
Hypotension
Faint heart sounds**
(& sometimes heart sounds in an unusual
location)

**How is tension pneumothorax
diagnosed?**

*Clinically!!!*
**(You are supposed to initiate treatment
*before* an X-ray is taken)**

**How is tension pneumothorax
treated?**

**Needle thoracostomy initially,**

**then**

**Chest tube (to water seal)**

**A proper lateral C-spine X-ray
must include what portions
of the spine?**

**C1 – T1**
(Top of T1, not necessarily the whole thing)

What position should the C-spine be
in when the lateral X-ray is taken?

Neutral

(Avoid hyperflexion or hyperextension)

If you suspect pneumothorax, but
can't see it on the chest X-ray,
what study should you order?

Exhalation chest X-ray

(this makes the pneumo bigger and easier
to see)

Why does a tension pneumothorax
get worse as time passes?

Air goes into the abnormal space, but
cannot escape, worsening the pressure on
normal structures with each breath

**In a tension pneumothorax,
what do you expect in terms
of pulsus paradoxus?**

**The patient should have it**

(not all of them do, of course)

**What *is* pulsus paradoxus?**

**Drop in systolic BP >10 mmHg during
inspiration**

**What is often noticed about the neck veins of patients with tension pneumothorax?**

**Distended neck veins**
(too much pressure for the blood to enter the atrium)

In tension pneumothorax, should the diaphragm on the affected side be high or low?

Low –
that side of the chest is full of air under pressure

In a tension pneumothorax, heart sounds are often distant, but the lungs are _____?

Hyperresonant
(more empty area than usual)

**If a tension pneumothorax causes tracheal deviation, which direction will the trachea go? Toward or away from the site of the tension pneumothorax?**

**The trachea moves away from the tension pneumothorax
(the pressure pushes it)**

What is the hallmark on EKG for pericardial tamponade?

QRS complexes that alternate between large amplitude and small amplitude

What is the special name for QRS complexes that alternate between large amplitude and small amplitude?

Electrical alternans

In electrical alternans, how much does the width of the QRS vary?

It doesn't –
only the amplitude varies

Supposedly, why does electrical alternans occur?

The heart is swinging back and forth through the fluid-filled pericardial sac

Aortic dissection due to trauma is associated with what types of fractures, especially?

1st or 2nd rib fractures

Aortic dissection due to trauma usually follows what type of injury?

Rapid deceleration

Traumatic aortic dissection usually begins at what anatomic location?

Between the ligamentum arteriosum & the left subclavian
(has to do with where the artery is "tethered")

What is the classic physical finding for aortic dissection?

BP is different in the two arms
(in reality, this finding is neither sensitive nor specific)

What findings on chest X-ray suggest aortic dissection?
(3)

1. Wider than normal mediastinum
2. Indistinct aortic knob
3. Esophageal deviation to the right

**If an aortic dissection patient develops a new heart murmur, what does this most likely indicate?**

**The dissection has gone backward and damaged the aortic valve**

**Neurological findings, particularly paralysis of one or both lower extremities, can be a presentation of aortic dissection. How?**

**The dissection has cut off circulation either to a limb, or to some of the arteries feeding the spinal cord**

Generally, what is the best way to diagnose aortic dissection?

CT with contrast
(TEE/US can also be used, but CT often gives more information faster)

**Rarely, an aortic dissection patient might also be hoarse. Why?**

**Pressure on the recurrent laryngeal nerve (it wraps around the ligamentum arteriosum on that side)**

**Rarely, an aortic dissection patient might present with neck swelling, ruddy complexion, and distended head & neck veins. Why?**

**Mass effect from the dissection creating SVC syndrome**

**What are the three categories you are checking when you use the Glasgow Coma Scale?**

1. **Eye opening**
2. **Motor response**
3. **Verbal response**

**How many points do you get on the Glasgow Coma Scale if you're dead?**

**Three**
**(There is no zero in the scale)**

**What is a perfect score on the Glasgow Coma Scale?**

**Fifteen**
**(Five per category)**

**If a patient with head trauma requires intubation, what medication are you supposed to give first?**

Lidocaine, 1 mg/kg
(It "blunts" the increase in ICP with laryngoscopy)

If you are doing a very brief trauma survey, you won't have time to do the Glasgow Coma Scale. What should you use instead?

AVPU evaluation
(The choices are:
A – alert
V – verbal but not totally alert
P – pain response
U – unresponsive)

Which three medications are most standard for rapid sequence intubation (RSI) in children?

Succinylcholine (short acting paralytic)

Atropine for children ≤1 year old
(bradycardia prevention)

An induction agent given before the paralytic (choices include etomidate, propofol, ketamine, thiopental, or fentanyl)

Which benzodiazepine medication was very commonly used in RSI, but is no longer recommended as a first line choice?

Midazolam (Versed®)
(onset too slow & potency too variable between individuals)

Atropine used to be given routinely to older children with RSI. Why is it used less now?

Data have not clearly supported its effectiveness in preventing bradycardia in children older than 1 year

Atropine is still definitely useful for reducing secretions

For which kids should atropine nearly always be used, if doing an RSI?

Those ≤1 year old

Consider in children <5 years old if succinylcholine will also be given

Following RSI, what medications need to be given, for patient safety & comfort?

A longer lasting paralytic –
Most often Rocuronium is used

&

Something for agitation/pain –
Most often fentanyl is used

Succinylcholine should not be used in which patients?

Burn & crush injury more than 24 h prior to intubation (the K+ takes time to rise)

Known or suspected hyperkalemia

Open globe injury (eye)

What alternative paralytic can be used in patients for whom succinylcholine is contraindicated?

Rocuronium

What is the main negative to using the alternative paralytic agent in RSI?

Much longer duration of action (if intubation unsuccessful, patient cannot breathe on his or her own for at least 30 min)

*(Note: a reversal agent has been developed called Sugammadex. It is in use in the EU, but not yet in the US)*

**Surgical cricothyroidotomy should not be done in children less than what age?**

**8 years**

**When should you choose a needle cricothyroidotomy, rather than a more definitive airway?**

**If you cannot intubate the trachea, and the bag-valve-mask technique is not working well** (for example, with significant orofacial trauma)

**Especially in a child, inability to obtain IV access should make you consider what other options?**

**Intraosseous or central venous access (intraosseous is usually quicker and better in kids)**

**If a patient is hypotensive, the first (and second) thing you should do to try to fix the pressure is _____?**

**Fluid boluses –**

**Give normal saline or lactated ringers**

**If you are treating a hypotensive pediatric patient, how should you "dose" the fluid resuscitation?**

**20 ccs per kilogram (can dose repeatedly)**

What must you watch out for if you use a central line to deliver fluids?
   (2)

1. Many central lines are long – the longer the tube, the slower the fluid flows
2. Many central lines have multiple lumens – more lumens mean smaller lumens, and this slows fluid delivery

**If a patient is hypotensive, is it acceptable to give pressors as a first response?**

**NO! Fill the tank *first!***
(Give fluids first)

**How much fluid should you give a hypotensive adolescent/adult, in general, when you are initially trying to correct hypotension?**

**One liter –**
**Okay to repeat**

(most trauma sources now recommend leaving the pressure a little low, rather than aggressively fluid resuscitating to normal BP)

If crystalloid does not correct hypotension, what type of fluid should be given next?

Blood – packed RBCs usually
(whole blood is also fine, but rarely used)

**Pain in the shoulder following trauma can sometimes be a sign of what abdominal problems?**

**Diaphragmatic irritation from blood in the belly**
**(or injury to the spleen or liver)**

**Shoulder pain that is really referred abdominal pain is called _____? (eponym)**

**Kehr's sign**

**Cullen's sign refers to what finding in the belly following trauma/intraperitoneal bleeding?**

**Ecchymosis around the umbilicus**

Grey-Turner's sign is another eponymic trauma sign. What is it?

Flank ecchymosis

(intraperitoneal or retroperitoneal bleeding)

Where are you supposed to look for ecchymosis related to abdominal trauma?

Flanks (Grey-Turner sign)

&

Umbilicus (Cullen's sign)

**What is the best diagnostic technique for evaluating abdominal trauma?**

**CT scan**
**(US FAST can be used as a "quick look" prior to more specific diagnosis)**

If, for some reason, CT scan is not available, and you suspect abdominal trauma, what other diagnostic modalities are available to you?

Ultrasound "FAST" scan (specific locations are checked for fluid – gives general but not very specific anatomic information)

&

Diagnostic peritoneal lavage (DPL)
*Rarely used, but sometimes still on exams*

What findings on DPL indicate that there is an abdominal injury?
(3)

1. Food/feces
2. >1,000 RBCs/cc
3. >10 ccs of free flowing blood

Adults & school-aged children usually develop traumatic diaphragmatic rupture on which side of the body?

Left

(in neonates, it is more common for diaphragms to rupture on the right)

How is a "myocardial contusion" treated?

Observation only, usually (antiarrhythmics can be used if needed – usually not necessary)

How is myocardial contusion usually diagnosed?

Abnormal wall motion (transient) on echocardiogram

How does a patient develop a myocardial contusion?

Blunt trauma to the chest

What is the main consequence of myocardial contusion?

Arrhythmia – but rarely significant (fortunately)

What is the most common sign of myocardial contusion?

Tachycardia

Splenic injury in children is usually managed in what way?

Non-operative (increasingly common in adults, too)

Although the spleen is the abdominal organ most often injured in <u>blunt</u> trauma, which is the organ most often injured in penetrating trauma?

The liver (it's the biggest abdominal organ, so it makes the biggest target)

| | |
|---|---|
| **How is traumatic liver injury usually managed?** | **Non-operative** (observation & supportive care) |
| Significant splenic and hepatic bleeding that requires intervention can sometimes still be managed nonsurgically. How? | Embolization |
| **Sudden cessation of the heart beat following trauma to the chest is called _____?** | **Commotio cordis/tardus** **(this medical term occurs as either cordis or tardus)** |
| **A child or adult hit in the chest with a ball, who suddenly drops to the ground, is suffering from _____?** | **Commotio cordis/commotion tardus (cessation of heart rhythm due to sudden mechanical impact)** |
| **Which children are at greatest risk for injuries from abuse?** (5) | 1. **Handicapped kids** 2. **Preemies** 3. **Children of young/overstressed or depressed parents** 4. **Multiple births** 5. **Parents were abused** |
| If one or more retinal hemorrhages are mentioned on physical exam in a vignette, without any other physical findings, what is the likely diagnosis? | Abuse (often from shaking) |
| **What kind of rib fracture is pathognomonic of child abuse?** | **Posterior** |
| **In terms of fractures, the overall pattern you expect to see in child abuse is _____?** | **Multiple fractures in multiple stages of healing** |
| **If something in the history or physical suggests child abuse, what radiology study do you need to order?** | "Skeletal survey" (X-ray the whole skeleton to look for old fractures) |

| | |
|---|---|
| **On head CT, what finding is pathognomonic for child abuse?** | **Interhemispheric subdural hematoma** |
| **Especially in very young children, what type of long bone fracture commonly occurs with abuse?** | **Metaphyseal corner fractures (aka "bucket-handle" fractures)** |
| For children older than 1 year, what type of fracture most often occurs with abuse? | Diaphyseal fractures (fractures of the middle of the bone – not the very end) |
| **Is a diaphyseal fracture pathognomonic for child abuse?** | **No – of course not (could have happened in a car accident, fall, etc.)** |
| **Is a metaphyseal corner fracture pathognomonic of child abuse?** | **Yes** (with rare exceptions) |
| **What aspects of the history should especially tip you off to investigate *possible* abuse?** | **If the story doesn't fit the injury** |
| **Are non-depressed skull fractures suggestive of child abuse?** | **Yes** (only suggestive, though – most will not be abuse) |
| **In terms of skin findings, what is most suggestive of child abuse? (3)** | 1. **Unusual burn patterns (perineal or stocking & glove patterns)** 2. **Linear injuries or other shapes consistent with a particular object** 3. **Multiple bruises, especially those not over bony prominences (not where you would expect them)** (judging the age of bruises is very difficult to estimate, so it is no longer recommended to look for bruises "in different stages of healing") |
| **If a child develops anogenital warts in the first year of life, what are the likely causes?** | **Abuse is possible, *but* perinatal acquisition of this common pathogen also occurs** |
| Are laryngeal papillomas suspicious for sexual abuse? | No – Usually acquired perinatally |

**Which STD is pathognomonic for sexual abuse?**

**Gonorrhea**

(Chlamydia is sometimes vertically transmitted from mother to child)

**What risk factor is *most associated* with physical abuse?**

**Family history of abuse**

**Round or wide linear bruises along the back may indicate what health practices seen mainly in Asian populations?**

**Cupping**

**Or**

**Coining**

**If a parent has used coin rubbing or cupping to treat his/her child, should you evaluate for abuse?**

**No –
It is a normal practice within certain cultures, and does not result in any significant harm**

**What is the leading cause of death in pediatrics and young adults?**

**Trauma
(mainly motor vehicle accidents)**

Trauma causes what proportion of pediatric deaths?

1/2

**What is the most common (general) cause of death for children in the first year of life, in developed nations?**

**Developmental & genetic conditions already present at birth**

What is the second most common cause of death for children ≤1 year old in developed nations?

SIDS (sudden infant death syndrome)

*(followed by prematurity & low birth weight-related conditions)*

What is the most common cause of death in the first year of life, worldwide?

Infectious disease
(especially due to pneumonia, diarrhea, & malaria, often complicated by decreased immune function due to malnutrition)

**What is the leading cause of death for children & young adults age 2–24 years, in North America?**

**Trauma**

**What are the other very common (general) causes of death for children 2–5 years old, in developed nations?**

**Developmental & genetic conditions already present at birth**

    &

**Cancer**

How is the pattern for likely causes of death different in the 5–14 year old group, compared to the 1–5 year old group?

They are the same except that the second & third most common causes reverse:

2–5 year olds:
Trauma
Developmental & genetic conditions present at birth
Cancer

5–14 year olds:
Trauma
Cancer
Developmental & genetic conditions present at birth

How is the pattern for general causes of death different for the oldest pediatric group, ages 15 & above in the US?

Trauma remains #1, followed by
Homicide – #2
Suicide – #3

**What is the most common lethal injury in pediatrics?**

**Head trauma**

When should you definitely *not* try nasotracheal intubation, based on patient injuries?

Same situations in which you shouldn't place an NG tube –

Significant orofacial trauma or Basilar skull fracture

    &

If the patient isn't breathing at all

Is nasotracheal intubation recommended in children who have not yet reached adolescence?

No

**Which fractures generally carry the biggest risk of severe blood loss?**

**Femur**

    &

**Pelvis**

**Which blood type is the universal blood donor?**

**O negative**
(It is okay to use O positive in an acute trauma setting, if that is the best answer choice available.)

What does "universal blood donor" mean?

This blood type doesn't generate an immune response in anyone

**What is the best early indicator of blood loss on physical exam in pediatrics?**

**Delayed capillary refill**
**(>2 s)**

When shouldn't you place an intraosseous line in a particular bone?

It's fractured

OR

an IO has already been attempted and placement failed (meaning the bone already has a hole in it from the attempted placement)

What complications do you worry about with intraosseous lines?
(4)

1. Infection (osteomyelitis)
2. Growth plate injury (angle away from it)
3. Fat emboli
4. Fluid leak/compartment syndrome

What sort of laryngoscope blade is usually recommended in pediatrics?

Straight (Miller)

How do you know how far to insert the ET tube?

3× the diameter of the tube
(gives you the number of centimeters from the lips)

How do you know how large of a tube you can use in small patients?

$$\frac{Age + 4}{4}$$

Which is more common in children, C-spine fractures or C-spine injuries?

Injuries

**What is it called if you have a spinal cord injury, but no fracture or other X-ray abnormality?**

**SCIWORA**
**(Spinal Cord Injury WithOut Radiological Abnormality)**

| | |
|---|---|
| If a patient is in a motor vehicle collision, and is not conscious upon arrival, but has no evidence of specific head trauma or injury, what is the likely explanation? | Axonal shear injury aka diffuse axonal injury– Common with rapid deceleration<br><br>(might get better, might not) |
| What is the 2-year mortality for undiagnosed child abuse? | >25 % |
| Does intracranial bleeding lead to hypotension? | No –<br>If anything, it tends to cause *hyper*tension, as a reaction to the bleed |
| What is "Cushing's response?" | Hypertension<br>Bradycardia<br>Apnea<br><br>In response to elevated ICP |
| Is Cushing's response (or reflex) usually seen early in the course of an intracranial bleed, or late? | Late (and it is not always seen at all) |
| Does scalp bleeding lead to hypotension? | Yes – bleeds profusely (especially in kids) |
| In addition to motor vehicle collisions and burns, what other types of trauma frequently cause pediatric injury & death? | Assaults<br>Falls<br>Bicycle related |
| If a pregnant Mom is injured, what is the guiding principle in taking care of the baby? | Resuscitate the Mom |
| If there is head trauma, what must you always remember to check? | The C-spine<br>(5 % will have a C-spine fracture!) |
| What is a contrecoup injury? | The part of the brain that gets hurt when it sloshes and hits the part of the skull *opposite the original impact* |
| **Which stuff dripping out of the head tells you that you might be dealing with a basilar skull fracture?** | **CSF –**<br>**Can drain from the nose (rhinorrhea) or the ear (otorrhea)** |

What unreliable test still sometimes appears on board exams, that is meant to tell you whether the fluid coming from someone's head is CSF or not?

The ring test –
Put a drop of the liquid on filter paper (or a sheet) and if a ring forms around the outside edge, it is supposed to be CSF

**If your head trauma patient has hemotympanum, how likely is it that he/she has a basilar skull fracture?**

**80 %**

**What other signs of bleeding on the face or head tells you to look for a basilar skull fracture?**
   **(2)**

**Battle's sign – blood over the mastoid
Raccoon eyes – blood around the orbit**

If you find a basilar skull fracture, what should you do about it?

Usually observe and alert neurosurgery –
(Antibiotics not useful)

If your trauma patient has rib fractures, what should you do?

If they are isolated fractures (not flail chest), give pain management

(Binding the area sometimes helps the pain, but is a risk for complications such as hypoventilation & pneumonia. You need to encourage deep breathing)

What is it important to give to a rib fracture patient, to encourage deep breathing, other than adequate pain management?

An incentive spirometer & instructions on how to use it!

(helps to prevent atelectasis & pneumonia)

What should you look for in any patient with a rib fracture?

Pneumothorax or pulmonary contusion

If a patient fractures a lower rib, what problems must you consider, in addition to lung issues?

Spleen or liver injury

Are rib fractures diagnosed by X-ray?

Diagnosis is clinical –
50 % will not show on X-ray

What is most worrisome about a sternal fracture?

It took a *lot* of force to do that (other structures may be damaged)

| | |
|---|---|
| Decreased breath sounds on the right, *dullness to percussion,* and respiratory distress combined with right sided blunt trauma suggests what diagnosis? | Hemothorax (patient may also be tachycardic/ hypotensive) |
| **A child is restrained in the rear seat in the rear seat with a lap belt only. A motor vehicle collision occurs. What fracture is this child at special risk to develop?** | **Chance fracture of the lumbar vertebra (unstable)** |
| **What intraabdominal injury is a child with a Chance fracture at unusually high risk for?** | **Perforated gut/viscus** |
| An adolescent is riding in the passenger seat with just the shoulder belt on. A frontal motor vehicle collision occurs. What intraabdominal injury is this child at special risk to develop? | Pancreatitis/pancreatic injury |
| **A child has a problem while riding his bike. He goes over the *handlebars*. What intraabdominal injuries should you be considering for this child? (2 main injuries)** | **Pancreatitis/pancreatic injury** & **Duodenal hematoma** |
| What urological exam findings should you be especially looking for in trauma? (3) | 1. Blood at the meatus 2. Perineal bruising 3. Boggy prostate (if age appropriate) |
| If any of the trauma urological exam signs is positive, what do you need to do next (assuming your patient is stable)? | Retrograde urethrogram – *Do not place foley until the urethra is confirmed to be intact!* |
| Which physical exam finding means you need radiological evaluation of the kidney (IVP, CT, etc.)? | Gross hematuria (Most injuries are minor & managed conservatively) |

| | |
|---|---|
| Bladder injury is usually associated with what sorts of trauma? | Penetrating<br><br>Or<br><br>Compression of the abdomen |
| Are you more likely to die of trauma in a city, or in a rural area? | Rural<br>(70 % of trauma fatalities are rural) |
| Your patient has an apparent spinal cord injury, and is hypotensive. What is the likely reason? | Neurogenic shock<br>(vasodilation in response to the sudden spinal cord injury)<br><br>• You should still look for other bleeding sources, of course! |
| **If your trauma patient can't feel anything below the belly button, where is the spinal cord lesion?** | **T10** |
| **The nipple line is approximately which dermatome?** | **T4** |
| How can you remember which dermatomes are at the nipple line and umbilicus level? | Imagine a patient who's a little heavy set sitting down – the waist line makes the mouth of a smiling face. The nipples above look like eyes.<br><br>Imagine the smiley face winking at you and saying: 10–4 Good buddy! |
| If your trauma patient can't feel anything below the clavicle, where is the spinal cord lesion? | C5 |
| There are two main groups of local anesthetics. What are they, and why is it important? | • Amides & esters<br>• If a patient is allergic to one, you can use an agent from the other group |
| How do you know which local anesthetics are in the same group? | Amides all have two "I's" in the generic name |
| When should you avoid combined lidocaine with epinephrine preparations, according to traditional teaching? | Areas at the edge of the body –<br>Digits, ears, penis, and end of nose<br><br>*(Current evidence supports the safety of lidocaine with epinephrine use in digits, & to some extent in other locations – but this is an area of transition, at the moment)* |

| | |
|---|---|
| What is the minimum acceptable urine output for a pediatric trauma patient? | 1 cc/kg |
| What is the minimum acceptable urine output for an adolescent/ young adult patient? | 0.5 cc/kg |
| What are the most common complications of large quantity blood transfusions?<br>    (3) | 1. Hypothermia (use a blood warmer)<br>2. Low platelets<br>3. Low factors 5 & 8 |
| **If a patient with a femur fracture suddenly decompensates, and goes into DIC, what happened?** | **Fat embolus**<br>**(from the long bone fracture) –**<br>**Very high mortality** |
| **What is the best overall study to evaluate for possible blunt abdominal injury?** | **CT scan –**<br>**With IV contrast & water soluble oral (or per NG) contrast, if possible** |
| **The brain has several different ways to herniate. One of the most common for patients who still might survive is called "uncal" herniation. What are the signs of uncal herniation?** | • *Dilated nonreactive pupil on same side (due to CN III compression)*<br>• **Central hypoventilation**<br>• **Contralateral hemiparesis** |
| **Closed head trauma that does not result in any bleeding or swelling, but still produces a temporary period of altered consciousness, or other cognitive changes, is called _____?** | **A concussion** |
| How many "grades" are there, when you are grading a concussion? | Three<br><br>Note: There are now several classification systems for concussions. Many clinicians have moved away from using the scoring systems, due to confusion about the best way to score them, and how useful the scoring really is. It may still be utilized on the boards, or by other clinicians with whom you speak, though. |

**If your patient lost consciousness due to a closed head injury, what grade of concussion are you dealing with?**

**Three**

**Following a concussion, how long must your patient avoid contact sports?**

**Until ALL symptoms, including any memory or concentration difficulties have completely resolved**

**What additional testing is often recommended prior to a return to contact sports, after a concussion?**

**"Provocative testing" –
Have the patient do an activity that increases BP & heart rate, such as sit-ups or jogging. Check whether any symptoms recur. IF SO, NO RETURN TO SPORTS YET**

**In both grades 1 and 2 concussions, the patient remains conscious. How are grades 1 and 2 different?**

**Grade 2 has amnesia for the event –
Grade 1 does not**

**What is a grade 1 concussion?**

**Transient confusion only**

How long must a grade 1 concussion patient sit out from contact sports?

No return to sports until symptoms completely resolve

&

Evaluated by a medical professional

**What are post-concussive symptoms?**

**Dizziness
Persistent headaches
Memory problems
Difficulty sleeping/concentrating
Sensitivity to light or noise
Depression, anxiety & fatigue**

**How long do symptoms from a concussion (also known as "mild traumatic brain injury" or MTBI) typically last?
(2 symptom categories)**

**Most have headache resolution within 2–4 weeks**

**Most have recovery of neuropsychological functions within 72 h**

**Why is it important to avoid a second closed head injury, if a concussion has recently occurred?**

**Increases likelihood of more serious neurological sequelae from apparently minor closed head injuries**

| | |
|---|---|
| **In addition to avoiding sports or other possible head injury, how should a concussion be treated?** | **Physical & cognitive rest!** |
| Which typical sports are high risk for MTBI (concussion)? | Boxing<br>Football/rugby/soccer<br>Ice hockey<br>Wrestling |
| Do concussion patients require evaluation at a medical facility? | Grades 2 & 3 do<br><br>(Grade 1 requires medical evaluation, but not necessarily at an institution) |
| **In a trauma patient, what is the "second C" of the ABC's?** | **C-spine**<br><br>**(Airway, breathing, circulation, C-spine)** |
| What does "tube & fingers in every orifice" refer to? | Trauma patient evaluation & management may require:<br>1. NG or orogastric tube<br>2. ET tube (possibly)<br>3. Foley (if no sign of urethral trauma)<br>4. Rectum checked for gross blood & tone<br>5. TMs checked for blood<br><br>*(Note: The need for routine rectal examination in trauma is currently an area of debate. Recent research suggests it may not be helpful & some clinicians now omit it.)* |
| Which patients are at especially high risk for hyperkalemia?<br>    (2 trauma-related;<br>2 condition related) | 1. Crush injuries/rhabdomyolysis<br>2. Burn patients<br>3. Renal failure<br>4. Dig toxicity patients |
| **Adults often suffer cardiopulmonary arrest due to a sudden cardiac event. What is the typical path to cardiopulmonary arrest in children?** | **Gradual deterioration – usually respiratory cause** |
| What type of medication is succinylcholine? | <u>Depolarizing</u> paralytic<br><br>(Depolarizing meaning it activates the muscles. It's the only depolarizing agent we use!) |

In children <5 years old, what premedication should you avoid giving, before administering succinylcholine?

A "defasciculating" dose of a non-depolarizing paralytic agent

(Very young children have insufficient muscle mass to cause significant ICP changes with fasiculations & some cases of bradycardia/asystole have occurred in very young children given a non-depolarizing agent combined with succinylcholine.)

How long does succinylcholine's effect last?

3–5 min (for most patients)

Succinylcholine should be avoided in patients who are thought to have what metabolic derangement?

Hyperkalemia

Is succinylcholine a reasonable choice for maintenance of paralysis? Why or why not?

No –
It lasts only for 3–5 min

&

Persistent depolarization of the muscles could be damaging & lead to other metabolic problems

What is the Sellick maneuver?

Gentle pressure on the larynx, toward the posterior neck, during intubation

What is the current status of the Sellick maneuver? Is it still recommended?

It is an area of controversy –
Was used to improve visualization of the larynx & to reduce reflux of gastric contents, but recent studies suggest it may not be helpful for either

Not recommended currently, but not clear what the final answer will be following further research

If the Sellick maneuver is in use, is it intended to prevent active reflux (vomiting)?

No –
Restricting vomiting can cause esophageal rupture!!!

What is ketamine's medication class?
What makes ketamine unique among this general class of medications?

- A dissociative anesthetic
- Essentially no respiratory depression

What situations is ketamine
especially good for, and why?
   (2 situations)

- Trauma – it increases BP
- Reactive airway patients – it
  bronchodilates

What respiratory problem can
occur with ketamine use?

Copious secretions – can give atropine first
to reduce them

Ketamine is great for most trauma
patients. Which trauma patients
specifically should not receive
ketamine, though?

Head trauma –
It increases ICP

*(this is now being debated, but for board
exams, avoid ketamine with head trauma)*

What annoying but not dangerous
ketamine side effect can limit its
use?

Emergence reactions/hallucinations –
most patients tolerate the drug well, though!

**What is the average heart
rate for school-aged children?**
(preschool & school-aged)

**80 beats per minute**

**What is a normal heart rate
for children 10 and older?**

**Same as adults –
about 75 beats per minute**

**What is the typical respiratory
rate for a preschooler?**

**Thirty**

**What is the typical respiratory
rate for a school-aged child?**

**Twenty-four
(double the adult rate)**

What is IV lidocaine used for?
   (2)

- Arrhythmia control
- To minimize the ↑ ICP that occurs with
  intubation (one-time dose)

Which other intervention is
important to minimize possible
increases in ICP, due to intubation?

Paralyzing the patient with succinylcholine
or a non-depolarizing paralytic agent before
intubation

*(this is probably the most important
preventative against increasing the ICP
with intubation – & is also important to
preventing multiple intubation attempts –
success is more likely when the patient is
paralyzed during intubation)*

| | |
|---|---|
| **What CNS manifestations would you expect in a very mild hemorrhage (class I – <15 %)?** | **Anxiety** |
| Severe hemorrhage (class 4 – ≥40 %) usually produces what sort of CNS changes? | Coma or at least deep lethargy |
| **What CNS manifestations do you expect to see with moderate hemorrhage (between 15 and 40 %)?** | **Irritable/confused/combative**<br><br>**Or**<br><br>**Lethargic (moderate)** |
| **How is the dose of epinephrine changed when you give it by ET (endotracheal tube)?** | **It is 10× larger**<br>**(Use 1:1,000 rather than 1:10,000 to keep the volume small)** |
| **What type of blood is given to children when transfusion is needed emergently, and type & cross is not ready?** | **O negative**<br><br>(O positive is alright, if O negative is not readily available) |
| How often can transfusion boluses be repeated? | Every 20–30 min is typical, but depends on the situation – more frequent is fine if needed |
| Why do opioids cause hypotension (mainly)? | They cause histamine release which dilates vessels |
| **How could you calculate the lower limit of systolic BP for children aged 1–10 years?** | **70 + (child's age in years × 2) = Minimum BP** |
| **How can you calculate the average or expected systolic BP for a child 10 years or less?** | **90 + (child's age × 2) = Expected BP** |
| **What is the normal respiratory rate for a toddler?** | **Thirty**<br>(same as a preschooler, just a different word) |
| **What is the typical heart rate for children 3 month to 2 years old?** | **About 100–130**<br>**(increasing age lowers heart rates)** |

At what level of hemorrhage will *central* pulses seem "thready?"

Severe
(Class 4)
(>40 % blood loss)

Capillary refill will slow down with what percentage of blood loss?

≥15 %
(Class 2 or worse)

**How many breaths should initially be given to a patient who is not breathing?**

**Two slow breaths**

(This has changed from earlier BLS protocols.)

**Which changes first in a pediatric patient in trouble – the capillary refill or the blood pressure?**

**Capillary refill slows**

**(heart rate will also increase before BP drops)**

# Chapter 3
# General Environmental Medicine Question and Answer Items

| | |
|---|---|
| What age group has the most prominent mammalian dive reflex? | Children |
| What is the mammalian dive reflex? (3 components) | 1. Bradycardia<br>2. Blood shunting to the CNS<br>3. Decreased metabolism |
| What is meant by "secondary drowning?" | Secondary drowning – Death by ARDS after a drowning incident |
| Is drowning in salt water better than drowning in freshwater? (likely to result in a better outcome) | No |
| When is a drowning patient most likely to develop ARDS? | 24–36 h after the incident |
| Can ARDS occur after a drowning, if the patient did *not* get any water in the lungs? | Yes (may be a type of neurogenic pulmonary edema – mechanism not clear) |
| **What is the main predictor of outcome in drowning?** | **Duration of immersion** |

© Springer Science+Business Media New York 2015
C.M. Houser, *Pediatric Tricky Topics, Volume 1*,
DOI 10.1007/978-1-4939-1859-1_3

**TV shows have made much of the potential to survive drowning if the water is cold enough. In general, drowning in a water temperature <6 °C has what implication for outcome?**

**Better prognosis than warm water drowning**

**(meaning resuscitation may be possible after a longer period of time in the cold water case)**

**Spectacular cases of survival after very prolonged submersion are occasionally reported. What is the typical pattern in these cases?**
**(3 important aspects)**

**Water temperatures are VERY cold**

**Often young children**

**The patient becomes rapidly hypothermic** *while still able to breathe,* **then submerged**

**Other than motor vehicle collision, the most common "accidental" cause of death in children is _____?**

**Drowning**

Middle, inner, and outer ear areas can be affected by barotraumas. Which is most serious?

Inner ear –
can produce *hearing loss* and vertigo/nausea/nystagmus

Is it alright for your patient with asthma to take scuba training?

Yes – IF the asthma is mild intermittent type

Other than psychosis, are there any psychiatric disorders that make scuba diving a bad idea?

Panic disorder

Should seizure disorder patients scuba dive?

Of course not!

If you are sending a patient on an air transport, and the patient has an ET tube or foley in place, what modification must you make to this equipment?

Fill with <u>water</u> not air
(Otherwise, the equipment is likely to fall out when the air expands and your balloons pop!)

How can you differentiate mild vs. severe hypothermia?

Severe has altered mental status
(mild has normal mental status)

What EKG wave is a buzzword for hypothermia? What does it look like?

- The Osborne or "J" wave
- An extra hump or slope on the down (right) side of the QRS

In a cold patient, is shivering a good or bad sign?

It is a *good sign* (normal heat generating response – also means that the patient is not terribly cold)

What two body systems are profoundly affected by cold, frequently leading to life-threatening complications?

1. The *heart* – highly prone to fatal arrhythmia when cold
2. The *blood* – all coagulation factors are temperature dependent (cold often produces or worsens DIC)

Are temperatures measured with a standard thermometer valid in a hypothermic or hyperthermic patient?

No – especially for cold patients, they are often not accurate.

(Use a specially calibrated thermometer with a rectal or other deep internal probe to get the "core" temp)

In a bradycardic, hypothermic patient, should you do CPR?

No –
If there is a pulse you should not do CPR. The mechanical stimulation can cause an arrhythmia

If your hypothermic patient is in V-fib, and you have shocked without success, what must you wait for before shocking again?

Core temp >85 °F

Should you perform CPR on a hypothermic patient in V-fib, while you wait for the temperature to rise?

Yes!

(CPR is avoided only if the patient has a perfusing heart beat – in a non-perfusing rhythm, some circulation is better than no circulation!)

What types of rewarming should you use for hypothermic patients?
(3 types)

First – Passive external
Second – Active external
Third – Active core

*(although none of it should interfere with resuscitation efforts)*

| | |
|---|---|
| What are passive external rewarming techniques? | Dry the patient<br>Remove wet clothes<br>Wrap in warm dry blankets<br>Heat lamps<br>(Same types of things you do in the delivery room!) |
| What are some active external rewarming techniques? | Warm $O_2$<br>Warm IV fluid<br>Forced convection (BAIR HUGGER blanket) |
| What are typical active <u>core</u> rewarming techniques? | Warm NG & foley lavage<br>Warm peritoneal lavage<br>(last ditch – fem-fem bypass or ECMO to rewarm blood externally) |
| If a hypothermic patient suddenly starts to generate an unusually large amount of urine output, it is called "cold diuresis." What transient kidney dysfunction causes cold diuresis? | Collecting duct failure to reabsorb water |
| Which patient groups are most at risk for hypothermia?<br>    (5 groups:<br>2 "accident" types<br>2 medical condition groups<br>1 medication-related) | 1. Burn patients (rapid loss)<br>2. Trauma patients (exposure)<br>3. Endocrine patients (hypothyroid & DM)<br>4. CNS & psychiatric patients (behavioral errors producing exposure)<br>5. Alcohol/sedative impaired |
| Now that Bretylium is not available, what is the drug of choice for arrhythmia in hypothermic patients? | Amiodarone |
| Regular defibrillation protocols cannot be followed for hypothermic patients. When can you repeat defibrillation, after the initial shock? | Core temp above 85 °F |

| | |
|---|---|
| What is "classic heat stroke?"<br><br>(5 attributes that make it classic) | 1. Epidemic (during a heat wave)<br>2. Nonexertional<br>3. Seen mainly in elderly & those with chronic disease<br>4. <u>Not sweating</u><br>5. Often causes death |
| There are two types of heat stroke. What are they called? | Classic & exertional |
| What makes exertional heat stroke different from classic heat stroke?<br>    (2 circumstances)<br>    (1 typical patient)<br>    (1 exam finding)<br>    (1 outcome) | 1. Exertional happens with exercise<br>2. Isolated case, not epidemic<br>3. Occurs in healthy young people<br>4. <u>Profuse sweating</u><br>5. Complications are common (but not usually permanent or severe) |
| What complications of heat stroke are most troublesome? | 1. CNS damage/seizures<br>2. Rhabdomyolysis (producing kidney failure)<br>3. DIC<br>4. Liver dysfunction (diffuse) |
| Why do cardiac disease and beta-blocker use contribute to heat illness? | Increased cardiac output is needed for increased heat loss |
| What is the difference between heat exhaustion and heat stroke? | <u>Heat exhaustion</u> presents with<br>• Nausea/vomiting/diarrhea<br>• Salt & water depletion<br>• Core temperature slightly elevated<br><br>Heat stroke = CNS dysfunction, severe core heat (>41 °C), death or permanent consequences common |

Amongst healthy patients, which ones are at especially high risk of heat illness while exercising?

- Those who cannot escape the heat
- Those who do not have adequate fluids available
- **_The very motivated (such as athletes)_**

What is the mainstay of treatment for heat stroke?

Evaporative cooling (fans & water)

What adjunct therapy can you use in heat stroke?

1. IV fluids (fluids have a lower temperature than the body temp)
2. Cool peritoneal lavage
3. Ice packs to groin & axillae
4. Extracorporeal cooling (fem-fem bypass)

Which cooling technique is thought to be more rapid in young, healthy patients of exertional heat stroke?

Cold water/ice water immersion

*This technique is often not practical in the healthcare setting, as patients cannot be properly monitored & resuscitated – it is also not recommended for other types of patients, as it may be physiologically too stressful & increase mortality!*

If you are treating a heat stroke patient, at approximately what temperature should you <u>stop</u> cooling the patient?

102 °F
(39 °C)

Why is it important to stop cooling your patient at a specific temperature?

Because the temp will continue to drop after cooling efforts end – and hypothermia worsens clotting problems

Are heat stroke patients uniformly dehydrated?

Not always
(can be a failure of thermal regulation, inability to sweat, etc.)

What medications increase the likelihood of heat illness?
(3)

1. Beta blockers (can't ↑ cardiac output!)
2. Anticholinergics (can't sweat)
3. Diuretics (can't sweat – less fluid)

| | |
|---|---|
| Why are pediatric patients are at increased risk for heat illness? | Heat loss mechanisms are not fully mature until puberty<br><br>*(also, like very elderly or ill patients, they may not be able to obtain fluids or seek cool shelter on their own)* |
| What are the other types of types of less serious heat illness? (<u>not</u> worrisome by themselves)<br><br>(4) | 1. Prickly heat (ruptured, blocked sweat gland)<br>2. Heat cramps (local Na shift)<br>3. Heat edema<br>4. Heat syncope (if nothing else about the syncope is suspicious) |
| If your patient's hands or feet swell during exposure to a hot environment, is there any cause for concern? | No –<br>It is a self-limited, normal cutaneous vasodilation. |
| What causes prickly heat rash? | Blocked sweat glands rupture → erythema and pruritis |
| What portions of the body usually develop prickly heat rash? | Clothed areas |
| Why do sweat glands become blocked in prickly heat? | The moist stratum corneum becomes macerated, and blocks the ducts |
| How is prickly heat treated? | Oatmeal baths & antihistamines (if needed) for pruritis |
| What is the main concern with prickly heat rash in children? | Superinfection from the itching (requiring antibiotic treatment) |
| How does "heat syncope" occur? | Dehydration + either heat vasodilation or low vasomotor tone for some other reason |
| How is heat syncope treated? | Rest<br>Remove from heat<br>IV & PO rehydration<br><br>*(remember to consider other causes of syncope, of course, before making the heat syncope diagnosis)* |

Five medication groups are especially likely to give you sunburn. What are the five groups?

1. Sulfas
2. Tetracyclines
3. Thiazides
4. Phenothiazines
5. Psoralens (used by dermatologists to create photosensitivity for psoriasis treatment)

What infectious agents are often found in burn wounds?

(one specific bug, one group of bugs)

1. Pseudomonas
2. GRAM negatives, in general

(of course, Staph & Strep species are also common)

Which burns require hospitalization?

1. Circumferential
2. Over a joint
3. Perineal burns
4. Significant facial burns
5. Dominant hand burns (if significant)

In the old burn classification system, there were 1st- through 4th-degree burns. What are the new levels, in the new system?

Superficial
Partial thickness
Full thickness
Complete

Describe a superficial burn? (2 aspects)

1. Red skin
2. No blisters

How deep does a superficial burn go?

Like it sounds –
Epidermis only (outermost layer)

How deep does a full-thickness burn go?

Significant damage to the dermis & often subcutaneous tissue –
Healing is via scar tissue & re-epithelialization

Describe a full-thickness burn?

White, waxy, no feeling, eschar

(Eschar is the special name for the tough tissue mass that results from deep burns)

What is a "complete" burn?

One that penetrates into the muscle, bone, or fascia beneath the skin

| | |
|---|---|
| How deep does a partial-thickness burn go? | Through the epidermis with some dermal damage *but* –<br>Enough dermis remains to allow full recovery (no scarring or limited function) |
| What does a partial-thickness burn look like? | 1. Red<br>2. Painful<br>3. Blisters |
| What is the difference in how a partial-thickness & full-thickness burn will heal? | Partial thickness –<br>No scar & no function problems<br><br>Full thickness –<br>Heals by scar formation<br>Function problems common |
| How can you guesstimate the body surface area (BSA) covered by a burn? | The patient's palm (without the fingers) is about 1 % of their body surface area |
| What is the "Parkland formula?" | The formula that allows you to calculate the fluid needs to a burn patient |
| How is the Parkland formula calculated? | 4 cc's × kg of pt weight × BSA burned = total ccs of fluid needed in 1st 24 h |
| How is the fluid calculated in the Parkland formula given? | ½ is given in the first 8 h *following the burn* (**not** *beginning when you started the IV drip*) –<br>The remainder is given over the next 16 h |
| How much body surface area does the trunk make up, in both adults and kids? | 36 %<br>(18 % back, and 18 % front) |
| How is the "rule of 9s" different for children? | Head = 18 %<br>(vs. 9 % adult)<br><br>Lower extremity = 14 % each<br>(vs. 18 % each in adolescents/adults) |
| The palm of the hand is equal to what percent BSA? (body surface area) | 1 %<br>(*this includes the palmar surface of the fingers!*) |
| After you have calculated the amount of fluid to be given to a burn patient, based on the Parkland formula, how do you divide it up when it is given? | Give half the total amount in the first 8 h following the burn –<br>Give the remainder over the 16 h left of the first 24 h post-burn. |

When might you want to give less fluid than recommended by the Parkland formula?

With inhalation injury (to decrease the likelihood of pulmonary edema)

- Adequate volume, though, is the main goal if you have to choose

Especially in a boards vignette, what should you be sure to investigate with a burn patient?

Whether he/she is also a trauma patient (e.g., has fractures due to jumping from a burning building)

How is that Parkland formula calculated?

4 ccs × kg of wt × % BSA burned = amount of fluid to infuse over the first 24 h

What physical findings or historical factors suggest inhalation injury in a fire?

1. Facial burns
2. Singed nasal hairs (aka vibrissa)
3. Sooty mouth
4. Fire in an enclosed space

Bees, wasps, ants, and hornets all belong to which insect class?

Hymenoptera

Which group of animals causes the most deaths per year? (choices include snakes, marine envenomations and bites, hymenoptera, cats, etc.)

Hymenoptera

If a patient has a serious allergic reaction to a hymenoptera sting, how fast does it usually progress?

50 % die within 30 min

Is it important to remove the stinger, in a hymenoptera envenomation?

Yes –
The longer it is in, the larger the venom load may be

(pinching & traction to remove it are both alright)

Where is the best place to inject an epinephrine autoinjector, for most patients?

The lateral thigh
(faster absorption than other sites, such as the arm)

Why are Africanized bees a bigger problem than the native species in North America & Europe?

They are much more easily annoyed, and attack with much more persistence, in larger groups

(significant ingestions are not uncommon, because the cloud of bees is quite thick)

| | |
|---|---|
| Are fire ant envenomations likely to cause serious allergic reactions? | Yes, it is a growing problem |
| What is the best way to manage local fire ant lesions? | Cool compresses<br>Topical anti-itch creams (e.g., low-dose cortisone)<br>Oral antihistamines |
| Are fire ants hymenoptera? | Yes – no wings, but hymenoptera |
| Do fire ants bite? | No –<br>They hold on with their mandibles so they can inject venom repeatedly via a sort of stylet on their abdomens |
| What second pathogen is often carried by ticks that transmit babesiosis? | Lyme disease<br>(patients may have both) |
| What is babesiosis? | A protozoal parasite infection, transmitted by ticks |
| What problems does babesiosis cause?<br>  (2) | 1. Anemia<br>2. Splenomegaly |
| What three treatments are useful in brown recluse spider bites? | 1. Cool compresses until the necrosis stops progressing (the damaging enzyme's activity is temperature dependent)<br>2. Hyperbaric oxygen (possibly)<br>3. Surgery (delayed)<br><br>*Note: Dapsone is no longer recommended due to lack of efficacy in studies, although still sometimes used. This is a change!* |
| What does a well-developed brown recluse bite look like? | A volcano (on the skin) |
| What is a buzzword for brown recluse spider bites? | (spreading) necrosis |
| Which spider has a dark violin shape on its top? | Brown recluse<br><br>Mnemonic:<br>Picture the brown recluse sitting by himself – a recluse – playing sad tunes on the violin |

| | |
|---|---|
| Should you use a tourniquet after a snakebite? | Generally – no |
| What two groups of poisonous snakes are found in the USA? | • Crotalids (pit vipers) & elapidae (coral snakes) |
| Which one is worse? | • Elapidae (coral snakes) |
| Is it a good idea to incise and suction snake venom from the wound after a snake bite? | No |
| Any hymenoptera sting creates a local reaction. For a patient who is <u>not</u> allergic to hymenoptera, how many stings are usually required to cause a toxic reaction? | More than 10 |
| What does a "toxic" reaction to hymenoptera consist of? (4) | 1. GI distress<br>2. Headache<br>3. Fever<br>4. Hypotension (sometimes) |
| Which poisonous spider has a "red hourglass?" | The black widow<br><br>Mnemonic:<br>Imagine a widow, dressed in black, watching the sands of an hourglass – or a widow with red lips and an hourglass shape! |
| Which of the two poisonous spiders behaves aggressively, and which one is shy? | Aggressive – black widow<br>Shy – brown recluse |
| Are scorpion stings dangerous? | Rarely – but severe effects are sometimes seen in small children (<6 years old)<br><br>*(In North America, scorpions dangerous to humans are found in the southwest, mainly Arizona – but may be found anywhere as pets, unwanted travelers, etc.)* |
| Which spider bite causes immediate pain, and sometimes causes (local) muscle rigidity? | The black widow |

| | |
|---|---|
| What two treatments are helpful for black widow bites? | • Antivenin<br>• Calcium (IV)<br><br>*(FYI – antivenin & antivenom are two acceptable ways to say the same thing)* |
| Are black widow bites serious? | Not usually |
| If a boards vignette describes a "painless" spider bite from a venomous spider, which spider was it? | Brown recluse (often initially painless) |
| Although neither brown recluse nor black widow bites are ordinarily life threatening, antivenin is available for which type of venom? | Black widow venom |
| If a boards vignette describes a recent bite or sting with a surrounding "pale" area, was it likely to be a spider bite or a scorpion sting? | Scorpion sting<br>(the venom has significant adrenergic vasoconstricting effects) |
| Electric shock or ice application to the site of a snake envenomation has been proposed as treatment modalities. What is the utility of each? | Shock – none<br><br>Ice – probably not helpful, and may cause a frostbite-type injury if used inappropriately in the field |
| **Is it a good idea to use a tourniquet to isolate the area a snake has bitten?** | **No – often causes more harm!** |
| What is a constriction band? | A close fitting bandage that impedes superficial venous & lymph flow |
| Is a constriction band a good idea in the case of snake envenomation? | Yes! – particularly if transit time to definitive care will be long |
| If a constriction band is used, how should it be placed? | Over the wound & extending 2–4 cm above the bite marks (meaning 2–4 cm closer to the heart) |

What proportion of bites from poisonous snakes is "dry?" (lack venom)

A significant proportion – Somewhere between 1/10 & >1/2 depending on type of snake & which study you read

Should you advise your patient or care givers to try to capture the snake that bit the patient?

Ah, no. Too much risk of further injury & delay.

Pain control is important for symptomatic envenomations. Which pain control medication class should you avoid in crotalid envenomations?

NSAIDs – may increase bleeding (which is already a problem, as the toxin also leads to coagulopathy & hematological problems)

Opiates are generally preferred

If you suspect a patient was bitten by a crotalid, but it seems to be a dry bite, should you send the patient home directly?

No, observe for 8 h – Symptoms sometimes take a little while to evolve

Under what circumstances should you give the antivenom CroFab®, following a crotalid envenomation?

If ANY signs of envenomation are present, give it

CroFab® is very well tolerated, and early administration may prevent damage that can have long-term sequelae

How is the amount of antivenom needed for a particular snake bite determined?

You can stop when: The clinical exam either improves or stops progressing, especially the swelling

Laboratory coagulation values improve

Systemic signs improve

As most snake bites occur on extremities, what is an important complication to monitor for?

Compartment syndrome (and infection, of course)

(Rhabdomyolysis can be an issue with rattlesnake envenomations, in particular)

Where can the rhyme, "red on yellow kill a fellow, red on black venom lack" be applied successfully (to decide whether a brightly colored snake might be poisonous)?

Only in the USA (coral snake)

If a patient is bitten by a coral snake, what local symptoms should you expect?

None initially

Sometimes a small local reaction develops later

If coral snake envenomation has occurred, when will systemic symptoms become evident?

Usually delayed – can be more than 12 h later, but then progress rapidly!

If coral snake envenomation is suspected, should you treat empirically?
Why or why not?

- Yes
- The symptoms are difficult to reverse once they appear, so prevention is better

What is the usual cause of death for coral snake envenomation?

Respiratory arrest/depression

Many of us think of coral snake bites as a problem just for scuba divers. Where else in the USA might a patient encounter a coral snake?

On land in Texas, Arizona, Arkansas. and some portions of the southeastern USA

Dog & cat bites that become infected are often polymicrobial. Other than typical skin flora microbes like Staph & Strep, which bacteria is most associated with infected dog & cat bites?

*Pasteurella multocida*

Aside from cleansing animal bites, what else should you do for the patient?
(3)

1. Debride the wound (if needed)
2. Consider giving Amoxicillin/clavulanate (PCN is a secondary option)
3. Give Td (tetanus) if needed

Which is more likely to become infected – dog or cat bites?

Cat

(Anywhere from 20 to 80 % depending on which study you read – Cat bites are more of a puncture wound.)

After an animal bite/attack, what should you <u>avoid</u> doing on the boards?

Closing the wound

(Note: This is an area of transition. In reality, we do often close for cosmesis. Mounting evidence shows that most bite wounds can be closed primarily with a <10 % infection rate & improved cosmesis.)

What type of bite is *most* likely to become infected?

Human bites

What is the pathogen most often associated with human bites?

*Eikenella corrodens*

After any bite injury, what must you check, in terms of vaccination issues?

1. Is the tetanus up to date (within **5** years if vaccination series is complete)
2. Is rabies vaccination & immunoglobulin needed?

Which patients should be given *tetanus* immunoglobulin?

(2 factors – they need to have both to get Ig!)

Ones who didn't have all three shots in the series (or you don't know whether they did)

&

Have more than a clean, minor wound

Neonatal tetanus is seen only in one circumstance. What is that?

Mom is not tetanus immune!

Do squirrels, rabbits, hares, or rodents carry rabies?

No

(They can acquire it, but generally don't transmit it – very rare case reports exist of transmission from pet rabbits in Southeast Asia, but this is exceptional)

We used to think that you had to be bitten to get rabies. Now we know it can also be acquired how?

Inhalation
(e.g. bat guano or urine – treat people who've been in an enclosed area with a bat)

| | |
|---|---|
| If rabies immunoglobulin is needed, how is it administered? | Amount is based on the patient's kgs |
| | & |
| | *all* Ig is injected at the site of the injury, if possible |
| | (for multiple bites, divide the dose & inject around the multiple sites) |
| If a patient needs rabies immunoglobulin, what else should also be given? | Rabies vaccine |
| Anytime you must give an immunoglobulin & a vaccine for the same disease (such as rabies or tetanus), what practical aspect should you always pay attention to? | Don't inject them at the same site! – The vaccine will bind the immunoglobulin!!! |
| What is the immunization regimen for rabies vaccination? | For immunocompetent patients, the CDC now recommends only four doses (although many experts disagree) on days 0, 3, 7, & 14 |
| | *This is a change!* |
| | Give it on days: 0, 3, 7, 14, & 28 *for immunocompromised (the old regimen)* |
| | Mnemonic: Once you get to day 7, just keep *doubling it* until you reach 1 month. |
| How is rabies treated, if infection develops? | Supportive only – virtually all die |
| | (coma induction technique has promise – but not a board topic) |
| What is the behavioral hallmark of rabies? | Hydrophobia (Fear of water – remember *Old Yeller*) |
| Salivation, or "foaming at the mouth," occurs during what stage of rabies infection? | Late – last stage (along with lacrimation and gait problems) |

| | |
|---|---|
| Muscle rigidity happens with tetanus. Does it also happen in rabies? | Yes – early stage (officially, stage 2 of 4) |
| Antivenin is occasionally needed for scorpion stings in what patient group? | Small children (<6 years old) |
| | *Note: Depending on the type of scorpion, and part of the world, antivenin can be required even for adults!!!* |
| What problem do scorpion stings occasionally cause in children (in the poisonous scorpion species Centruroides found in the southwest USA)? | Seizure-like motor activity, but the patient is fully aware |
| Why is it a bad idea to wash jelly fish-stung areas (same for anemones) in water? | Plain water will cause automatic discharge of the stinging units (even from a dead jellyfish) |
| How do nerve gases work? | They are acetylcholinesterase inhibitors |
| | (producing SLUDG symptoms – Salivation Lacrimation Urination Defecation GI distress) |
| Is it possible to be poisoned by nerve agents while treating patients who have been poisoned? | Yes – only with certain agents, though (mainly VX) |
| | (usually absorbed through skin) |
| What is the initial treatment for nerve agent poisoning? | • Atropine |
| What is the follow-up treatment for nerve agent poisoning? | • Pralidoxime (aka 2-PAM) |
| Why is a follow-up treatment needed for some types of cholinergic poisoning? | Some poisons form covalent (permanent) bonds over time, making treatment difficult – pralidoxime prevents the bonding |

What is the special danger of treating victims of nerve agent attack?

Contamination of health care workers (from the patients, themselves) is more likely than in other CBRNe scenarios.

(CBRNe = chemical, biological, radiological, nuclear, & explosive)

What is the correct initial decontamination procedure for unknown exposures?
(gases, microbes, etc.)

Soap & water
(whole body and hair should be cleansed)

*Remove all contaminated clothing & other personal items, of course.*

If a patient is contaminated with radiation, should healthcare workers be concerned about possible radiation contamination to them while caring for the patient?

Generally not

In additional to soap & water decontamination, what additional measures are recommended with nuclear exposure?

Trim the nails & hair
(removes some additional sources of radiation)

Which type of radiation is known to be dangerous – ionizing or non-ionizing?

Ionizing

Which cells are most vulnerable to gamma radiation?

Lymphocytes

When is the best time to check the lymphocyte count, in order to give a prognosis, after radiation exposure?

48 h

Mild radiation poisoning produces what effects?

Nausea & vomiting for 1–2 days

What are three ways to "guesstimate" the level of radiation exposure?

1. Skin – if it's erythematous, then the dose was high
2. Lymphocyte count at 48 h
3. Interval to symptoms – shorter is worse

| | |
|---|---|
| If you suspect that a patient has either pulmonary anthrax, or pulmonary plague, what drug can you give that will treat both? | Doxycycline |
| The drug of choice for a known anthrax infection is? | Ciprofloxacin (also in children) |
| Both plague and anthrax have a much milder type of disease than the pulmonary form. Which forms are these? | Cutaneous anthrax  &  Local plague infection (skin & nodes, bubonic plague) |
| The "mild" form of anthrax has a particular appearance. What is it? | Looks like a black eschar (black burned area) |
| Is this "mild" anthrax form still dangerous? | Yes – due to risk that it will become systemic (at least 20 % do so without prompt treatment) |
| Which type of electrical injury is usually worse, AC or DC? | AC (alternating cycles in the tissue) |
| Which tissues have the most resistance to electrical current? | • Tendon & bone |
| Which have the least? | • Nerve & blood |
| Why is it important to know how much resistance a tissue has to electrical current? | The current will lose more heat into the tissues with more resistance – this causes more damage to these tissues |
| In an electrical burn, which determines the damage more – current or voltage? | Current |
| If a child bites on an electrical cord, and is now fine – aside from burn wounds at the margin of the mouth – what dangerous delayed effect can occur? | Bleeding from the nearby labial arteries. This can take up to 2 weeks to occur (with rare case reports of longer). |

What special instructions must you give to the parents or caregivers for a child with margin of the mouth burn wounds, prior to discharging the child?

Explain the risk of delayed bleeding & management with direct pressure

If a patient is not directly struck by lightning, but is affected by lightning striking nearby, what is that called?

Lightning splash

Do lightning splash patients require any treatment or evaluation?

TMs should be checked
(rupture is common with lightning)

CPK sent to check for any rhabdomyolysis

EKG is usually performed (but not terribly useful)

What is the most important principle in resuscitation after a lightning injury?

Rescue breathing must continue
*(Pulse will often return spontaneously!)*

Prolonged exposure to a wet, cold, environment tends to cause what famous disorder?

Trench foot
(a la WWI soldiers in trenches)

When trench foot rewarms, how will it present?

Dry, red, and very painful to the touch
+/− edema and bullae

How is trench foot treated?

Rewarm, then keep the foot warm, dry, and elevated
(and pain management)

How do you treat a frostbitten, or possibly frostbitten, extremity?

Rapid rewarming in 41 °C water

*Do not begin rewarming, though, if the area cannot be kept warm! Warming & cooling phases, for example during transport, are worse than waiting longer for warming!*

What is a good cutaneous clue as to whether frostbite is deep vs. superficial?

The skin blebs are clear in superficial, and hemorrhagic in deep

| | |
|---|---|
| What is the main significance of distinguishing deep from superficial frostbite? | Deep results in permanent and significant tissue loss<br>(Superficial only damages tissues that can regrow.) |
| Chilblains are treated much like trench foot. What are "chilblains?" | Painful inflammatory skin lesions (usually heal well) |
| What causes chilblains? | Intermittent exposure to cold, damp, air (not freezing temperature air, and not actual exposure to liquid – just damp cold air) |
| What causes trench foot? | Long-term exposure to a wet and cold (but not freezing) environment |
| Both chilblains and trench foot are treated with _____ & _____? | Elevation & rewarming |
| Because trench foot only develops with submersion in a wet environment, it usually occurs on the foot. Chilblains are likely to occur where? | Any exposed surface |
| Which organs are most often damaged in any type of blast incident? | Hollow organs (including TMs – rupture & lungs – pneumothorax) |
| In an explosion, which four organs are most likely to suffer damage from the blast itself? | – Ear (TM rupture and ossicle damage)<br>– GI (ruptured viscus)<br>– Lung (pneumothorax or air emboli)<br>– CNS (concussion or air emboli) |
| Which patients *do not* need any treatment after possible tetanus exposure? | <5 years since last tetanus |
| If a patient sustains a "clean" wound, and had a tetanus immunization 6–10 years ago, is any treatment required? | No –<br>Within 10 years is alright for clean wounds |

If a patient sustains a "dirty wound," how do you know whether a tetanus booster is needed?

If it is <u>more than 5 years</u> from the child's most recent booster (or original immunization) a booster is needed

**In addition to obviously dirty wounds, what three other important categories of wounds are considered to be dirty?**

1. **Crush injuries**
2. **Burns**
3. **Frostbite**

If a child has a "clean" wound, how do you know whether a tetanus booster is required?

>10 years since last immunization

What is the significance of calling the tetanus immunization for older people Td, and the one for younger people DT (DTaP)?

Vaccines listed as DT have 10 times the amount of diphtheria toxoid as do the Td vaccines
(same stuff, just different proportions)

**At what point do you switch to a Td formulation, rather than a DT vaccine formulation?**

**>7 years old**

(after that, there is a much greater probability of bad reactions to the diphtheria part, so the amount is kept low)

Pertussis outbreaks have been a problem in recent years. What change in immunization protocol addresses this problem?

Addition of a pertussis immunization with tetanus immunization in adolescence

(age 11 years or older, 11–12 years old preferred – may be given later in life, is no pertussis immunization administered ≥11 years old)

# Chapter 4
# General Toxicology Question and Answer Items

| | |
|---|---|
| **How effective are "gastric emptying" techniques? (stomach pumping, ipecac, etc.)** | **50 % (or less) of material removed <u>if</u> used within 1 h** |
| **In the past, ipecac was recommended as part of every family's first aid medicine kit. Is it considered a good idea for non-medical personnel to administer ipecac?** | **No –** <br> **It is RARELY indicated, and when it is, that needs to be under medical direction (preferably poison control)** <br><br> **It is used in the prehospital phase of care ONLY!** |
| **When is it acceptable to use ipecac, in terms of the ingestion?** <br> **(6 conditions)** | 1. **Ingestion has serious risk of morbidity or mortality** <br> 2. **Patient is far away from medical care (>1 h transport time)** <br> 3. **Large, recent ingestion (<30 min before administration)** <br> 4. **Substance not bound by charcoal** <br> 5. **Plant ingestion** <br> 6. **Not a hydrocarbon or caustic (you don't want to bring those up again, causing more damage to the structures they pass)** <br><br> *(Note: Ipecac has become SO unpopular that many practitioners think it should never be used. That is not the case, although circumstances for its use are quite limited.)* |

© Springer Science+Business Media New York 2015
C.M. Houser, *Pediatric Tricky Topics, Volume 1*,
DOI 10.1007/978-1-4939-1859-1_4

| | |
|---|---|
| **When is it acceptable to use ipecac, in terms of the patient's characteristics?** | **Patient must be capable of protecting the airway & not have any GI contraindications to inducing vomiting** |

**If you give ipecac, what should you expect to happen?**

1. **Delayed emesis (15–20 min)**
2. **Prolonged emesis (not one or two bouts!) mainly over the first hour**

**When is ipecac completely contraindicated?**
**(1 material item; 3 patient items)**

1. **Material is toxic if it comes back up (caustics, hydrocarbons)**
2. **Patient not protecting airway (seizing, not alert)**
3. **Patient <6 months old**
4. **Bleeding disorder (risk of Mallory-Weiss tear in the stomach from repeated emesis)**

When is "gastric lavage" a reasonable choice?
(2)

1. Recent ingestion of a life-threatening agent (<1 h is best)
2. Charcoal can't bind the agent

(Note: "To teach the patient not to try that again" is not the answer on the boards! or in real life!)

When should you definitely not use gastric lavage?
(3)

1. Caustics & Hydrocarbons (worse to bring them up than to let them sit)
2. Unprotected airway
3. Nontoxic agents, of course

To decrease the risk of complications during gastric lavage, how is the patient positioned?

Left lateral decubitus & head 20° downward

**When is whole bowel irrigation worth trying?**
**(4)**

1. **Sustained release pill ingestion (large)**
2. **Iron, lithium, or lead**
3. **Transdermal patch ingestion (whole patch)**
4. **Drug packers (can also be removed surgically)**

When you give the first dose of charcoal in a multi-dose charcoal treatment, what should you consider ordering with it, for an adolescent patient?

A cathartic – usually sorbitol

*Note: Not recommended in young children, due to risk of dehydration and/or electrolyte imbalance, & lack of proven efficacy in improving GI issues or the toxic ingestion itself*

Should you order a cathartic with each dose of charcoal (if you are using multidosing)?

No
(can cause dehydration & electrolyte problems in patients of any age)

Does a single dose of charcoal produce constipation?

No

(only seen with multidosing regimens)

**What is a normal osmolal gap?**

**Less than 10**

**What are the typical toxins & molecules that produce osmolal gaps?**

**Alcohols, antifreeze, & ketones**

**1. Ethanol**
**2. Acetone**
**3. Isopropanol**
**4. Ethylene glycol**
**5. Methanol**
**6. Ketoacidosis**

**How do you calculate the patients osmolality (roughly)?**

**2× Na + 10**

(good rough estimate if BUN and glucose are near normal limits)

How do you calculate the patient's osmolality precisely?

$$2Na + \frac{BUN}{2.8} + \frac{Glucose}{18} + \frac{ETOH}{4.6}$$

How can you calculate the osmolal gap?

Measured osmolality – calculated osmolality

($\geq 10$ is abnormal)

**Why do we care about the osmolal gap?**

**It suggests the patient has:**

**1. ketones**
**2. antifreeze (a type of alcohol)**
**3. or some other sort of alcohol on board**

Which one is sometimes useful in toxic ingestions – urine acidification or alkalinization?

Alkalinization

(acidification is a distractor answer – not currently used)

Why is changing the urine's pH sometimes a useful strategy?

Certain molecules are "trapped" in the renal tubules with the change in charge, and cannot return to the bloodstream

What three toxins are especially good candidates for urine alkalinization treatment?

1. Aspirin/salicylates
2. INH
3. Phenobarbitol

How is charcoal dosed?

1 g/kg to maximum of 100 g

**In general, when is multi-dose charcoal useful?**
   **(2)**

1. **Sustained release preparations**
2. **Hepatically recirculated meds**

**Name some common or important overdose medications that you would want to use multi-dose charcoal with.**
   **(4)**

1. **Theophylline**
2. **Phenobarbital**
3. **Carbamazepine**
4. **Salicylates**

**When is charcoal <u>not</u> useful in a toxic ingestion?**
   **(4 cases:**
**2 patient related**
**2 item related)**

1. **Metals (e.g., lithium, iron)**
2. **Caustics, alkali/acid**
3. **Ileus**
4. **Obstruction**

**When is charcoal specifically contraindicated?**

For GI reasons:

1. **Caustics (not useful & obscures endoscopy view)**
2. **Ileus**
3. **Obstruction**

What is a <u>normal</u> anion gap?

Less than 13

How is anion gap calculated?

$(Na) - (Cl + CO_2) = gap$

(positive electrolyte minus negative electrolytes)

**The MUDPILES mnemonic goes with anion gap acidosis – What do the letters stand for?**

**Methanol, metformin**
**Uremia**
**DKA**
**Paraldehyde**
**Iron & INH**
**Lactic acidosis**
**Ethylene glycol**
**Salicylates**

(For lactic acidosis, think of CO or CN as possible causes in tox questions)

How can you remember which anion gap mnemonic is which?

NAGs (non-anion gap) are HARD UP. Therefore MUDPILES must go with anion gap acidosis.

**What is the antidote for a calcium channel blocker overdose?**
**(2)**

**1. Calcium**
**2. Glucagon**

**What is the antidote for a β-blocker overdose?**

**Glucagon**
**(isoproterenol is also a possibility)**

**In a coumadin overdose, what is your first choice to correct coagulation parameters?**

**FFP**
**(Fresh Frozen Plasma)**

Vitamin K will _not_ correct the bleeding problem fast enough – FFP supplies the missing factors right away!

Vitamin K is also listed as an antidote for coumadin (warfarin) toxicity. What are the problems with vitamin K use?
(2)

1. Unreliable onset of effect & always delayed
2. Can be difficult to regulate later if the patient needs ongoing anticoagulation

**On the boards, should you give both FFP & vitamin K for warfarin toxicity?**

**Yes –**
**If there is an answer choice with both, it is usually correct**

How do patients end up overdosing on warfarin?
(4)

1. Iatrogenic – level gets too high on med regimen
2. Medication dosing errors
3. Child gets hold of med
4. Rat poison

If your patient has ingested rat or mouse poison, what should you watch for, in addition to anticoagulant effects?

If it was the "wheat pellet" sort of poison, it may also contain a CNS depressant (alphachloralose)

Charcoal will bind it

Household detergents come in three classes – what are they & which one is dangerous?

Cationic, anionic, and non-ionic

Generally, only cationic is dangerous

If a patient eats or drinks a household detergent, what is the main toxic effect you should be worried about?

Corrosion of the gastric tissue (or in some cases respiratory tissue), due to the detergent's pH – typically the bases are the biggest problem

If a child has eaten a toxic plant, what should you do?

Give charcoal – it binds most plant toxins

There are many potentially toxic plants in the world. What are the typical effects of toxic plant ingestion?
 (3 categories)

• Nearly all produce gastric irritation, usually with nausea/vomiting/diarrhea
• Many also produce CNS depression & sometimes seizures, if the ingestion is large enough
• Some produce arrhythmia

Unintentional toxic ingestions are most common in which age group?

Young children <6 years old

(Toddlers & infants are especially inquisitive!)

Unintentional nicotine ingestion is especially common in which pediatric age group?

<1 year old!
(70 % of nicotine ingestions are in this group)

What sorts of tobacco products are most often ingested by children?

#1 is cigarettes
#2 is smokeless tobaccos
(meaning snuff or chewing tobacco)

Electronic or "e-cigarettes" are relatively new. Is there a risk of an e-cigarette toxic ingestion?

Yes –
The fluid used to fill them can be consumed

The labeling on an e-cigarette or its fluid indicates its nicotine content. How should you interpret the milligrams listed?

The milligrams listed are PER CC!

(So if it says 16 mg, that means 16 mg nicotine PER cc!)

What does of nicotine is thought to be the minimum lethal dose for pediatric consumption?

1 mg/kg

(recent evidence suggests that significantly higher amounts can likely be tolerated)

What aspect of liquid nicotine ("vaping") products *should* limit their ingestion?

Nicotine is quite irritating to the mucosal surfaces

*(but some of the fluids have flavoring which may make them more attractive)*

In addition to the nicotine content, are there other toxins you should worry about in a vaping fluid ingestion?

Yes, they often contain highly toxic alcohols & essential oils –
Content varies, but more consistency is likely as regulation of e-cigarettes increases

How do large nicotine ingestions cause death, generally?

"Nicotinic" stimulation leads to respiratory muscle paralysis & death –

Acetylcholine receptors of the nicotinic sort are overstimulated. When the muscle can no longer respond, it is effectively paralyzed & breathing ceases

After ingesting a small quantity of nicotine, what effects would you expect?

Tachycardia & vomiting

With a moderate nicotine ingestion, what effects are typical?

Ataxia & seizure

*(ataxia is a somewhat unusual toxicological effect, so good to remember)*

At higher doses, what is special about the nicotine toxidrome?

Nicotine activates both nicotinic & muscarinic ACh receptors, causing both sorts of effects!

(SLUDGE is added to the nicotinic effects)

**TCA overdose and sympathomimetic overdose look very similar – how can you tell them apart?**

**TCAs are anticholinergic – <u>no sweating!</u>**

| | |
|---|---|
| **Please recite the "anticholinergic mantra."** | *Hot as hell* (fever)<br>*Blind as a bat* (dilated, can't accommodate)<br>*Dry as a bone* (can't sweat)<br>*Red as a beet* (skin flushing)<br>*Mad as a hatter* (cognitive & psychotic changes)<br>*Bloated as a bladder* (urinary retention & decreased gut motility)<br>*Seizing like a squirrel!*<br>(seizures not uncommon) |
| **How do you recognize the "cholinergic toxidrome?"**<br>(4) | 1. **The gut moves like crazy (emesis & diarrhea)**<br>2. **Everything runs (salivation, urination, defecation, lacrimation, bronchorrhea)**<br>3. **Bradycardia**<br>4. **Miosis (small pupils)**<br><br>Remember, this toxidrome is the *opposite* of the anticholinergic toxidrome. |
| **What makes the cholinergic toxidrome dangerous, rather than just annoying?** | **The typical toxidrome symptoms are *muscarinic*, <u>but</u> the nicotinic system is also affected →**<br>**seizures, muscle twitching and/or weakness leading to <u>respiratory failure</u>** |
| **What agents typically cause cholinergic poisoning?**<br>(3) | 1. **Insecticides (carbamates & organophosphates)**<br>2. **Certain mushrooms**<br>3. **Nerve gas agents** |
| How can you remember that cholinergic poisoning critically involves the nicotinic receptor? | Insecticides that gave the bug SLUDGE would give you an unhappy bug, but probably not a <u>dead</u> bug<br><br>(SLUDGE is salvation, lacrimation, urination, defecation, GI distress/emesis) |
| How do most cholinergic toxins produce their effects? | They mess up the enzyme that normally breaks down ACh (acetylcholinesterase), so too much is constantly available |
| **What is the first line antidote for any kind of cholinergic poisoning?** | **Atropine** |

| | |
|---|---|
| **Why is atropine helpful?** | **It is a competitive inhibitor of ACh, so binds to the same sites, without producing a response. This reduces the percent of molecules bound to a receptor that produce a response (allowing muscle cells to recuperate)** |
| | *(Remember, though, that atropine only binds at muscarinic ACh sites!)* |
| **What type of poisoning needs 2-PAM (pralidoxime) treatment?** | **For organophosphate-type poisonings** |
| Why is it important to give pralidoxime in organophosphate-type poisonings? | If it is not given promptly, the AChase is permanently disabled (referred to as "aging") |
| | (This means your patient will not recover until the body has synthesized all new AChase.) |
| How do the chemical nerve agents, a possible agent in chemical terrorism incidents & of course war, work? | The same way as the insecticide poisonings – acetylcholinesterase is inactivated, producing both muscarinic & nicotinic effects |
| If a nerve agent is inhaled, how long will it take to work (in general)? | Not long! Seconds to minutes |
| How long is required before nerve agent effects are seen, if the agent is absorbed from the skin? | Hours – anywhere from about 2–18 h |
| If nerve agents are acetylcholinesterase inhibitors, then what is the first line of treatment? | Atropine & pralidoxime (to prevent chemical aging) |
| As a healthcare worker, do you need to worry about contact with the patient poisoning you, if the patient has been exposed to a nerve agent by breathing it? | Generally not – Nerve agent vapors generally dissipate rapidly on their own – VX present on the skin might still be an issue |
| | (simple decontamination with soap & water will remove liquid nerve agent present on the skin) |

| | |
|---|---|
| Which nerve agent remains in the environment & is a hazard long after the initial release? | VX<br><br>(the others dissipate rapidly) |
| A chemical agent that causes severe pain & irritation of the skin, eyes, & mucous membranes, with respiratory problems & blister formation following those effects, is likely to be from what class of agents? | Vesicants or blistering agents |
| What are some examples of chemical agents that cause this skin & respiratory presentation? | Mustard gases (there are several types)<br>Phosgene (famous for its odor of "freshly mown hay")<br>Lewisite |
| Are vesicant/blistering agents a contact hazard for healthcare workers? | Yes – decontamination should be performed<br><br>*(both to remove the agent from the patient & to prevent contamination of others)* |
| Do vesicant agents stay in the environment, creating an ongoing risk to others who go there? | Yes<br><br>(like the nerve agent VX) |
| In general terms, how do these blistering agents work? | They form acids on the skin or other bodily surfaces, generating damage |
| What is special about the eye effects of vesicant/blistering agents? | Corneal damage occurs regularly |
| Other than decontamination, how do you treat a patient exposed to a blistering agent? | Supportive care & burn-type protocols may be required |
| Are blistering agents generally persistent in the area where they were released? | Yes –<br>& that means they are also a risk to healthcare workers until the patient is decontaminated |

Some chemical agents act primarily via the lungs, and are called choking or suffocating agents. Some of these are also a concern in industrial accidents. What are the most typical agents in this category?
(4)

Chlorine gas

Hydrogen chloride

Phosgene (also a vesicant/blistering agent)

Nitrogen oxides

Other than irritation to musical & skin surfaces, what are the main effects seen after a choking agent exposure?

Dyspnea & cough

Wheezing & bronchospasm

What is the main mechanism of action for the choking agents?

They are acids or acid formers when in contact with mucosal surfaces – these agents have most of their effects in the respiratory tree, though

Is recovery usually complete if the patient survives a choking agent exposure?

No – chronic respiratory difficulties often follow significant exposures

How is a choking agent exposure treated?

After removal from environment & provision of oxygen – supportive care

How do tear gas & pepper spray affect people?

VERY painful to eyes & makes seeing (temporarily) difficult

(they also react with water to form irritating compounds on mucosal surfaces, especially the eyes)

Are long-term effects expected from an exposure to lacrimation agents (tear gas & pepper spray)?

Generally not

Which chemical agent can be delivered in many different ways, and shuts down cellular protein synthesis?

Ricin
(from castor beans – made famous by espionage assassinations carried out this way)

Do protein synthesis inhibiting agents remain in the environment after release?

Only briefly

| | |
|---|---|
| What is the usual result of ricin ingestion? | GI symptoms with gut hemorrhage, Followed by liver & kidney failure |
| What is the usual result of ricin inhalation or injection? | Flu-like illness in the first day, then – inhalation form presents with pulmonary symptoms first |
| | injection form tends to go directly to multisystem organ failure |
| How is ricin exposure treated? | Supportive only – With significant exposure, high mortality regardless of care |
| In general, for any patient suspected of being exposed to a chemical agent, what should be done prior to the patient entering the healthcare facility? | Simple decontamination – Remove clothing & wash with soap & water *(this removes the majority of most agents that do not dissipate on their own)* |
| Which bizarre chemical agent presents with ataxia & anticholinergic effects, sometimes including mass shared hallucinations? | BZ also known as Agent 15 – It is an "incapacitating agent" because most individuals will not become very ill from the exposure, but the ataxia & cognitive impairment renders them unable to take effective action |
| What is the mechanism of this odd chemical agent? | It is anticholinergic in both peripheral & central *muscarinic* neurons, causing delirium & peripheral effects |
| Is this anticholinergic agent a contact threat for the healthcare personnel? | Yes! It is very persistent!!! *(It is quite potent, and lasts more than 4 weeks in the soil)* |
| How should BZ or Agent 15 be decontaminated? | The usual way – Remove cloth, wash with soap & water (particulate matter can be gently brushed away) |
| Is BZ dangerous in any way? | Yes, two ways – Patients are a danger to themselves through bizarre behavior (be sure that no weapons are available) |
| | & |
| | Hyperthermia is common |

If anticholinergic effects are the problem in BZ intoxication, is it wise to give a medication like physostigmine (a cholinesterase inhibitor) to increase acetylcholine?

Generally not – too many serious side effects (including cardiac arrest)

*(It may be used for intractable seizures, tachycardia or agitation not responding to other measures, with caution.)*

For control of agitation & bizarre behavior, what medication is recommended in BZ intoxication?

Benzodiazepines

Which common plant ingestions also cause anticholinergic delirium?
    (3)

Jimsonweed

Belladonna

Nightshade

**What is the antidote to opiate overdose?**

**Narcan™ (aka naloxone)**

**What is the "typical" finding in opiate overdose (pupils)?**

**Pinpoint**

**(meperidine may dilate)**

What opiate source might be in the family medicine cabinet & not considered dangerous by the family?

Lomotil™ (Diphenoxylate)

**What are the dangers of opiate overdose?**

**Apnea!** (& some hypotension – not usually bad except in young children)

**Acute toxic effects from the extrapyramidal system are typically seen with which medications?**

**Antipsychotics (haldol, droperidol, etc.)**

**&**

**Thiazines**

**What two medications can be used to treat extrapyramidal toxic effects?**

1. **Diphenhydramine (Benadryl™)**
2. **Benztropine (Cogentin™)**

**What are the symptoms & signs of extrapyramidal toxicity?**

1. **Dystonic reaction (oculogyric crisis & torticollis)**
2. **Akathisia (need to move)**
3. **Rigidity**
4. **Dysphagia**
5. *Laryngospasm*

How is a sedative/hypnotic overdose treated?

Supportive care
(and make sure that is the only drug onboard!)

**Should you use flumazenil to reverse a sedative/hypnotic overdose?**

**No – could cause tough to control seizures**

What two general categories of medications make up the majority of sedative/hypnotic medications?

Benzodiazepines

&

Barbiturates

**Is isolated benzodiazepine or barbiturate overdose dangerous?**

**Generally not – monitor BP and respiratory rate (apnea occurs with ETOH & other medication combinations)**

How is ETOH withdrawal treated, in terms of medications?

Benzodiazpines

&

Clonidine

**Why is it important to treat ETOH withdrawal?**

**Autonomic instability can be dangerous**

**In addition to ETOH, what other withdrawal syndromes must be treated?**
    **(4)**

1. **Benzos**
2. **Barbiturates**
3. **Cocaine**
4. Clonidine

Amphetamines, cocaine, and PCP all belong to what general medication class?

Sympathomimetics

**In general, what is the presentation of someone overdosing on a sympathomimetic?**

**Like someone having an obvious m.i. – (anxious, sweaty, tachycardic, hypertensive, dilated pupils)**

**What medication counteracts the effects of sympathomimetics?**

**A benzodiazepine**

| | |
|---|---|
| In addition to m.i.-like findings, what other problems may accompany sympathomimetic overdose? (2) | Seizures & Hyperthermia |
| **In mg/kg, how much Tylenol™ (aka acetaminophen, paracetamol, or APAP) will prove toxic?** | **140 mg/kg (about 10 g in an adult)** |
| **What is the antidote for acetaminophen toxic ingestions?** | **NAC (n-acetyl cysteine aka mucomyst)** |
| What is the loading dose for NAC? | 140 mg/kg (same as the toxic dose of APAP) |
| For patients who cannot tolerate or have contraindications to oral treatment with NAC, what other treatment option do you have? | Administer IV Known as the "British Protocol" – 150 mg/kg over 60 min then 12.5 mg/kg/h for 4 h then 6.25 mg/kg/h for 16 h (total treatment time 21 h) |
| **In an APAP ingestion of unknown quantity, how do you know whether APAP will reach toxic levels?** | **Check the serum APAP level *at 4 h* & compare to chart** (The chart is also called a "nomogram." In the case of APAP, the Rumack-Matthew nomogram is the name of the one used.) |
| Should a higher than usual dose of NAC be given, if charcoal is also given at the same time? | No – *this is a change from previous practice!* (Activated charcoal does adsorb some of the NAC, but the impact is so small, that no adjustment is needed.) |
| After the loading dose, how is NAC dosed? | 70 mg/kg × *17 doses* Given 4 h apart (There is a new NAC formulation that makes the infusion regimen simpler) |
| **What patient group is <u>least likely</u> to develop liver toxicity with APAP?** | **Young children** |

Why is NAC helpful in APAP overdose?

It provides a glutathione-like substance that binds the toxin

**What are the stages of APAP toxicity?**

1. **GI symptoms which resolve spontaneously, then**
2. **Liver & renal dysfunction**
3. **↑ LFTs & GI symptoms return**
4. **Recovery or liver failure**

Why is too much APAP (acetaminophen) toxic?

The liver can only detoxify so much APAP at a time – excess amounts saturate glutathione and kill liver cells

**Why is ethanol toxicity more dangerous in kids than adults?**

**It can produce rapid hypoglycemia**

**(immature liver – limited glycogen stores)**

**Why is ETOH withdrawal dangerous?**

**Autonomic dysregulation (fever, tachycardia, HTN)**

**When do the potentially dangerous complications of alcohol withdrawal begin?**

**Typically 2–3 days** *after the last drink!*

What are the dangerous features of alcohol withdrawal collectively referred to as?

DTs
(delirium tremens)

Why are alcoholic patients given "banana bags" of vitamins, thiamine, folate, & magnesium?

In an effort to prevent Wernicke-Korsakoff syndrome

(caused by dietary deficiencies common in alcoholics)

What medication class is primarily used to treat ETOH withdrawal?

Benzos!

What are the stages of ETOH withdrawal?

1. "Shakes" – tremor & agitation
2. Hallucinations
3. "Rum fits" – seizures
4. DTs – autonomic dysregulation (significant mortality)

**"Disk hyperemia" on funduscopic exam is a buzzword for toxicity from what substance?**

**Methanol**

Mnemonic:
Picture a red "disk" of methanol being tossed like a Frisbee at a party, and splashing on the players' eyes when they grab it, producing tunnel vision!

What are the four treatment choices for methanol ingestion?

1. 50 % ETOH (IV if possible)
2. Folate (cofactor)
3. Fomepizole
4. Hemodialysis

Fomepizole can be used for which two toxic ingestions?

The two that can be treated with ETOH – Ethylene glycol

&

Methanol

**A patient who appears to be *drunk*, but complains of *visual symptoms* is probably suffering from what ingestion?**

**Methanol**

Methanol intoxication patients are especially likely to complain of what visual symptom?

Tunnel vision
(then blindness)

What makes methanol toxic?
(2 reasons)

1. It is a CNS depressant (like ethanol)
2. It forms a toxic metabolite – formic acid

*(the formic acid is responsible for the hallmark features of methanol toxicity)*

In addition to visual complaints, what other signs may be evident in methanol toxicity?
(4)

1. Seizure
2. GI complaints
3. Abdominal pain/pancreatitis
4. Respiratory distress

Large ingestions of either methanol or ethylene glycol may require what more invasive sort of treatment?

Hemodialysis

The toxic effects of methanol are decreased by what IV therapy?

Bicarb –
Improves pH & may decrease both visual symptoms & active forms of formic acid

What else can you give, to enhance recovery from methanol toxicity?

Folic acid or folinic acid –
Increases rate of formic acid (toxic metabolite) breakdown

If someone drinks isopropyl (rubbing) alcohol, what two organ systems will be primarily affected?

1. CNS (intoxication/CNS depression, cerebellar signs & coma possible)
2. GI (hemorrhagic gastritis)

Which other two organ systems are sometimes affected in isopropanol ingestions (rubbing alcohol)

Pulmonary (pulmonary edema)

&

Cardiovascular (hypotension)

Why is it especially important to know about isopropanol toxicity?

It is the most common toxic exposure in the USA

(probably because it is so accessible, especially now that isopropyl-based hand sanitizers are so popular!)

**What are the "classic" lab findings with isopropyl alcohol ingestion?**

1. **Ketosis (from the acetone produced)**
2. *No acidosis*
3. ↑ **osmolal gap**

How is a very significant isopropyl alcohol ingestion treated?

Supportive care + hemodialysis

(hemodialysis is thought to increase elimination of both the acetone metabolite & isopropanol

A child ingests a common household product. The child is ill appearing, has an osmolal gap, but is *not acidotic*. What is the likely ingestion?

Isopropyl alcohol

(treat with supportive care, proton pump inhibitors may be helpful for gastritis)

How is a severe ETOH intoxication treated?

Respiratory & BP support
(supportive care)

Severe cases of toxic alcohol ingestions can all be treated with what technique?

Hemo*dialysis*

Mnemonic:
Think of the alcohol evaporating through the dialysis membrane.

Ethylene glycol is most commonly found in antifreeze – what other common liquids may also contain it?
(2)

Paint

&

Solvents

What are the treatment options for ethylene glycol ingestion?
(3)

1. Fomepizole
2. IV or PO ETOH
3. Dialysis

(ETOH is *a lot* cheaper than fomepizole, and readily available(!), but fomepizole has a better side-effect profile)

**If a vignette involves a liquid ingestion and urine findings, what is the likely ingestion?**

**Ethylene glycol**

**Specific urine findings are:**

**1. RBCs**
**2. Fluoresces**
**3. "Envelope" shaped crystals**

Are there any cofactors that might be helpful in treating an ethylene glycol ingestion?

Yes –
Giving thiamine (B1) & pyridoxine (B6) speeds processing of toxic metabolites to less toxic forms

**Why are β-blockers not recommended for cocaine overdose (or exposure to an unknown sympatho-mimetic)?**

**Unopposed alpha activity could result – causing vascular contraction & ischemia**

**Why is unopposed alpha activity a bad thing?**

**Ischemia/infarction –**

**Alpha activity constricts arterial blood delivery – Beta-blockade decreases the amount of blood the arterial system tries to deliver.**

**Antihistamine overdose looks the same as what other medication toxidrome?**

**Anticholinergics**

**(including many aspects of tricyclic antidepressant overdose)**

**If a patient seems to have anticholinergic poisoning, but also has a widened QRS, what toxic ingestion is likely?**

**Tricyclic antidepressant**

**(QRS > 100 ms is wide)**

If patients with antihistamine/anticholinergic ingestions become agitated, what medication can be used?

Any benzodiazepine

Physostigmine inhibits acetylcholinesterase. Should you use it with anticholinergic toxidromes?

No –

Risk of seizure & *asystole*

(Use in consultation with a toxicologist only.)

What patient populations are likely to have arsenic poisoning?

Attempted suicides
Attempted homicides
Immigrants from 3rd-world nations
(due to contaminated well water)

**If you need to test for arsenic exposure, how do you do it?**

**Urine level (24-h)**

   **or**

**X-ray if ingested**

*(Blood level is not useful)*

How do patients accidentally encounter arsenic?
   (3)

1. Pesticides/herbicides
2. Soil
3. "Alternative" medications

**What is the antidote for arsenic toxicity?**
   **(2 options)**

**BAL (British anti-Lewisite)**

**(Penicillamine is also used)**

Mnemonic:
Have a BAL with arsenic!

Generally speaking, why is arsenic toxic?

Reduces ATP

| | |
|---|---|
| What are the effects of chronic arsenic poisoning? | *Neuropathy & diarrhea*<br>Paresthesias in limbs<br>Hyperkeratotic or hyperpigmented rash |
| **What derm-related finding is a buzzword for arsenic toxicity?** | **Mees lines – seen in chronic or subacute poisoning**<br><br>*(white opaque lines in the nails – of course other things can also cause them, but not in a tox vignette!)* |
| What is the classic presentation of an acute arsenic ingestion? | Metallic taste in the mouth<br><br>&<br><br>Dysphagia |
| What are the most common effects of acute arsenic poisoning?<br>(2 systems) | 1. GI – N/V/D & abdominal pain<br>2. Cardiovascular issues (arrhythmia, vasodilation, and capillary leakiness) |
| **What is the antidote for heparin overdose?** | **Protamine sulfate**<br>(1 mg/kg) |
| Where might a child or suicidal patient find warfarin?<br>(2) | 1. Medication bottles<br>2. Rat poison |
| **What hematological abnormality goes with warfarin toxicity?** | **Prolonged PT** |
| **In a barbiturate overdose, what physical exam finding is a bad prognostic sign?** | **Cutaneous bullae** |
| Is urine alkalinization useful in barbiturate overdose? | Yes |
| Barbiturates used in medicine generally produce hypotension & CNS depression. What barbiturate variant has the opposite effect? | Methaqualone |
| Most treatments for β-blocker and calcium channel blocker toxicity are the same. Which is unique to calcium channel blockers? | Calcium IV<br>(makes sense!) |

| | |
|---|---|
| What treatment options can be used in both β-blocker and calcium channel blocker toxicity? | 1. Fluids<br>2. Catecholamines (usually those with both alpha & beta effects)<br>3. Pacemaker<br>4. Glucagon (short term) |
| Overdose of most typical antiseizure medications results in what classic triad of signs & symptoms? | Dizziness<br>Ataxia<br>Nystagmus |
| With severe overdoses of antiseizure medications, what signs/symptoms are likely? | Coma<br>Seizure (paradoxically)<br>Arrhythmia |
| For small ingestions of valproate, what sort of care is usually needed? | Activated charcoal (single dose) if recent<br><br>Supportive care |
| What are your options for treating really large overdoses of valproate? (2 decontamination techniques, 1 quantity reduction, 2 medications) | 1. Activated charcoal<br>2. Whole-bowel irrigation, mainly for extended-release formulations<br>3. Hemodialysis<br>4. Naloxone (sometimes improves level of consciousness – mechanism unclear)<br>5. L-carnitine (a cofactor) |
| What role does L-carnitine play in valproate processing? | It is often low in overdose or chronic valproate use (multiple mechanisms)<br><br>&<br><br>It is needed for mitochondrial energy production & valproate processing +<br>It is needed to reduce ammonia levels by restoring mitochondrial urea processing |
| What are the main ways you treat a carbamazepine overdose? (4 items – decontamination, seizure control, cardiovascular effects controls) | MULTIdose-activated charcoal (unusual in pediatrics)<br><br>Benzos for seizures<br><br>Bicarb for QRS > 100 ms<br><br>Supportive care, including fluid support for hypotension |

What unusual decontamination measure should be considered for a large ingestion of extended release carbamazepine pills?

Whole-bowel irrigation (closely monitor electrolytes, but risks of toxicity can outweigh the risks of the irrigation)

Why does carbamazepine have effects on the cardiovascular system?

Like phenytoin, it is a sodium channel blocker

Can arsenic toxicity be treated?

Yes (Chelation with BAL or penicillamine)

**What is the leading cause of toxin-related death in the USA?**

**Carbon monoxide**

**How is carbon monoxide poisoning treated?**

**100 % oxygen**

**&**

**Hyperbaric oxygen** (if needed & available)

**If a group of people living in the same household all have vague flu-like symptoms that improve during the day (while at work or school), what is the diagnosis?**

**Carbon monoxide poisoning**

(usually from home heating systems or sometimes from poorly maintained space heaters)

**At what time of year is carbon monoxide poisoning most common?**

**Fall – when heating systems are first turned back on**

**Which patients are at special risk from CO poisoning?**

**Those with high $O_2$ consumption – fetuses, very young children, pregnant women**

**Does CO cross the placenta?**

**Yes – and it's very fond of fetal hemoglobin!**

**What is the point of treating CO poisoning with $O_2$?**

**It reduces the half-life of carbon monoxide**

**What are the symptoms of carbon monoxide poisoning?**

**Headache**
**Nausea**
**Confusion**

| In severe CO poisoning, the patient may be comatose or seizing. Why? | The underlying problem is hypoxia – hypoxic patients seize and become comatose |

**How is carbon monoxide poisoning definitely diagnosed?**

**Blood level of carboxyhemoglobin needed – Treatment should be started based on clinical findings & suspicions**

What does the ABG of a CO poisoning patient usually show?

*Often normal!* –
The problem is that the O2 bound to hemoglobin is very low –
the ABG doesn't measure this

**Will the pulse ox help you evaluate CO poisoning patients?**

**No.**

Why are pulse ox readings often misleading with CO poisoning patients?

The pulse ox is looking for percentage of hemoglobin that is saturated –
CO saturates hemoglobin very nicely!

(just not with the right molecule)

Although the carboxyhemoglobin level is helpful for diagnosis and management of CO poisoning, how well does the level correlate with toxicity?

Not well

(Treat the patient, not the number.)

What types of products cause "caustic ingestions?"

Acids & alkalis

Which type of caustic ingestion is more common – acid or alkali?

Alkali

**Which type of caustic ingestion usually causes more damage?**

**Alkali**

(causes liquefactive necrosis)

**How is the damage done by a caustic ingestion evaluated?**
**(2)**

**1. Upright CXR (to evaluate lungs & see free air)**
**2. Endoscopy**

Should steroids be given routinely for caustic ingestions?

No –
Steroids *were* used previously, depending on endoscopy findings *but are no longer recommended*

| | |
|---|---|
| Although recommendations vary, if a boards vignette suggests diluting a caustic ingestion (with water), is that alright? | Generally not<br><br>(opinions vary on this, but depending on the substance, risks generally outweigh possible benefits) |
| **Overdose with what cardiac medication presents like opiate overdose?** | **Clonidine** |
| What are the four main CNS effects of clonidine overdose? | Lethargy<br>Apnea<br>Miosis<br>Depressed reflexes<br>(much like opiates) |
| What kind of a drug is clonidine, generally speaking? | Alpha agonist |
| What cardiac effects does clonidine have, in overdose?<br>(3) | 1. Bradycardia<br>2. Hypotension<br>3. A-V block |
| In clonidine overdose, what medication may be helpful in reducing at least some of the effects? | Naloxone |
| The two common sources of carbon monoxide poisoning are _____ & _____ ? | • Home heating<br>• Fires |
| What is the underlying pathophysiology of cyanide poisoning? | Anoxia<br><br>(the oxygen based energy systems of the cell are shut down) |
| The most common source of cyanide toxicity is _____ ? | Smoke inhalation<br><br>(burning plastic gives off cyanide) |
| **The characteristic odor your patient is supposed to have if he or she is cyanide poisoned is _____ ?** | **Bitter almond** |

**The characteristic color of the blood, mentioned in carbon monoxide poisoning is _____?**

**Cherry red (bright red)**

How does cyanide poisoning present?

Very rapidly –
Nausea & abdominal pain
Coma
Cardiovascular collapse

If cyanide toxicity is suspected, how is it treated (the general idea)?

By creating methemoglobinemia

(Cyanide likes methemoglobin more than it likes normal cells.)

Specifically, how is cyanide toxicity treated?
  (3)

With the cyanide kit:
1. Amyl nitrite (inhaled before IV access established)
2. Sodium nitrite IV
3. Sodium thiosulfate IV

Which plants contain digitalis?

Foxglove

&

Oleander

Digitalis overdose causes what three main problems?

1. AV block
2. Arrhythmia
3. Hyperkalemia

**How does digitalis work?**

**It inhibits the Na-K ATPase pump**

**How is digoxin overdose treated?**

**Digibind (antibodies to digoxin) binds the drug**

**What electrolyte problem significantly worsens the toxicity of digitalis overdose?**

**Low potassium!**

**Should calcium be given to hyperkalemic patients on dig? Why or why not?**

**NO! –**

1. **The hyperkalemia could be a symptom of dig overdose, rather than real elevated K**
2. **Giving calcium with high dig level could theoretically "freeze" the heart in contraction**

What is a tetanically contracted heart, due to digoxin and excess calcium, called?

"Stone heart"

For an adult-sized patient with an unknown amount of digoxin ingested, how much Digibind (Dig Fab fragment) should you give?

5–10 vials usually

If the amount of dig ingested *is known*, how can you calculate how much Fab fragment is needed?

$$\frac{\text{Serum dig level} \times \text{weight}}{100} \text{ equals}$$

the number of vials to use

To treat a dig overdose, the main number you would like to know is _____?

Serum dig level

(assuming the tablets were not *just* eaten, and sitting in the gut as you treat!)

**Although a variety of arrhythmias occur with dig toxicity, which one is considered to be pathognomonic for it?**

**PAT (paroxysmal atrial tachycardia) with AV block**

What does PAT with AV block mean?

The atria go through episodes of rapid firing, but most are not conducted to the ventricles

What is the *most common* dysrhythmia observed with dig overdose?

PVCs

(premature ventricular contractions)

In the setting of dig overdose, what potassium level tells you to start Fab fragments right away?

5.5

(Kind of high for anyone, definitely high if dig is also on board!)

All this stuff about dig overdose and potassium is confusing.
So high is bad and so is low?

- High is bad because it indicates a more severe poisoning
- Low is bad because it indicates there will be more toxicity of whatever dig was ingested (or given)

Bradycardia often occurs with dig overdose. Can you use atropine to treat it?

Yes

What other medications can be helpful in managing the cardiovascular aspects of dig overdose?
(2)

Magnesium
*(for SVT, do not use with bradycardia or block)*

&

Phenytoin

**Which antiarrhythmic class is *contraindicated* in dig overdose?**

**Class 1a antiarrhythmics**

**(too much sodium channel effect –** examples are quinidine & procainamide)

Phenytoin also has sodium channel effects. Why is it alright to use it in digitalis toxicity?

Phenytoin eliminates the tendency of dig to produce arrhythmias, *while keeping the inotropic improvements*

Phenytoin has also been shown to be more effective than lidocaine at ending dig-induced SVTs

A patient on hallucinogens usually presents similarly to what type of overdose?

Sympathomimetics

(tachy, anxious, dilated pupils, hyperthermic)

How does hallucinogen use present differently from sympathomimetic overdose?

Psychosis!

How are hallucinogen patients treated?

Sedation, haldol, wait for it to wear off

**What are the main problems with hydrocarbon use/abuse?**

**1. Pulmonary irritation**
**2. Arrhythmia**

How do hydrocarbons put the heart at risk for arrhythmia?

They make the myocardium oversensitive to other stimulation
(much like hypothermia)

**What type of hydrocarbon use typically puts the myocardium at risk for arrhythmias?**

**Sniffing**

&

**Huffing**

**A patient is picked up by EMS in a life-threatening arrhythmia. Some cans were found near the victim, who apparently collapsed when some security guards chased the group out of their location. What happened?**

**A group was huffing –**

**The sudden catecholamine burst put this patient's heart into a non-perfusing rhythm**

**What common PALS/ACLS drug must not be used with hydrocarbon patients in dysrhythmia?**

Epinephrine

(it makes it worse)

If the chest X-ray initially looks good following a hydrocarbon ingestion, how reassuring is that?

Not very –
Chest x-ray needed six hours later due to frequent delay in findings

What physical aspects of hydrocarbons increase their likelihood of causing problems?
  (3)

↑ volatility
↓ surface tension
↓ viscosity

How can you remember which physical aspects of hydrocarbon make them dangerous?

They are all things that make it easier for the HC to get into the lungs
(even if it's already in the stomach)

What aspects of their chemical makeup render some hydrocarbons more dangerous than others?

Halogenation (e.g., PVCs, carbon tetrachloride)

  &

Aromatic hydrocarbons
(ring structures)

Generally, hydrocarbons should not be lavaged, because it increases their potential contact time with the lungs. In what situations might lavage of hydrocarbons be alright?

1. Large quantity
2. Very toxic (pesticide, leaded gas, halogenated or aromatic)

**What is the antidote to INH toxicity?**

**B6
(pyridoxine)**

**Seizures in a pediatric patient, that are not responding well to the usual medications, could be due to an accidental ingestion of _____?**

INH

What is the usual presentation of an INH overdose?
  (2 components)

1. Seizures or coma
2. Metabolic acidosis (anion gap)

Unexplained and difficult to manage seizures in the right population could always be _____?

INH overdose
(immigrants, children, prisoners, etc.)

**What is the most common, but also least lethal, form of poisoning?**

**Plant ingestion**

Pulmonary edema, not from a cardiac cause, is associated with what types of poisonings?
  (4)

M methadone &
  meprobamate
*O opiates*
P phenobarbital
*S salicylates*

Mnemonic:
You need MOPS for the lungs with these poisonings.

**Mydriasis goes with which general toxin groups?**
  **(4)**

**Antihistamines**
**Antidepressants**
**Anticholinergics**
**Sympathomimetics**

Hypoventilation goes with "slow" breathing. What drugs or toxins tend to cause hypoventilation?

S sedative hypnotics
L liquor
O opiates
W weed (marijuana)

**Vesicles & bullae are sometimes seen with what toxins/meds?**
**(not including weapons)**

**Barbiturates**
**Sedative hypnotics**
**CO**

Blue skin can indicate cyanosis <u>or</u> what tox-related condition?

Methemoglobinemia

Which reasonably common substances tend to cause methemoglobinemia?

Nitrates/nitrites
Aniline dyes
Dapsone
Phenazopyridine

(Phenazopyridine is the drug used for symptomatic relief of UTIs – turns the urine bright orange)

Bright red skin or blood is supposed to go along with which toxicity?

CO

In addition to many children & pregnant women, which other patients need hyperbaric oxygen after carbon monoxide exposure?

Those with CNS or cardiac toxicity

Whole bowel irrigation can be considered for tox patients in what situations?
   (3)

1. Body packer (packets not ruptured)
2. Sustained released medication
3. Charcoal can't bind the toxin

(assuming the nurses really like you!)

Multi-dose charcoal is a good idea for what four common groups of medications?

1. Sustained release
2. Salicylates
3. Phenobarb
   (due to enterohepatic recirculation)
4. Theophylline

**What toxic substances can usually be seen on X-ray?**
   (5 groups – The mnemonic spells COINS, which you can also see on X-ray!)

**C chloral hydrate &
   cocaine packets
O Opiates
I iron & other heavy
   metals
N neuroleptic agents
S sustained release &
   enteric coated pills**

If you want to find out whether a patient has been exposed to a toxin *in the last few days,* what is the best test to send?

Urine
(toxins are cleared from the blood much more rapidly)

| | |
|---|---|
| How do methemoglobinemia patients present? (2) | Like hypoxic patients Or Just cyanosis |
| How is methemoglobinemia treated? | Methylene blue fixes it |
| What is the problem in methemoglobinemia? | The iron becomes too oxidized to carry oxygen |
| Will methemoglobinemia improve if you give oxygen? | No |
| **What color is the blood in methemoglobinemia?** | **"Chocolate brown"** |
| **Will pulse ox readings help you to evaluate a patient's oxygen state if he or she has methemoglobinemia?** | **Not really –** **The abnormal Hgb state makes the pulse ox unreliable** |
| Why does methylene blue work as a treatment for methemoglobinemia? | It puts the iron back to its usual state, so it can carry oxygen again |
| In what situations is mercury toxic? | Inhaled or injected |
| **Is mercury from a thermometer toxic?** | **Not unless it's inhaled** |
| Which body systems does mercury toxicity affect? | CNS GI Renal |
| How is mercury poisoning treated? | Chelation (with BAL or succimer) |
| **What is the main action of MAO inhibitors?** | **They block degradation of catecholamines** |
| **What are the symptoms of MAO inhibitor toxicity?** | **HTN Headache Tachycardia** |

**Foods containing large amounts of what substance can cause a hypertensive crisis for patients taking even normal doses of MAO inhibitors?**

Tyramine
(aged cheeses, wine, fava beans)

What medication class, when combined with an MAOI, can produce a hypertensive crisis?

Amphetamines

**Which two common medications can cause a "hyperpyrexic syndrome" or "hyperthermic syndrome" if combined with an MAOI?**

**Meperidine (Demerol)**

**&**

**Dextromethorphan**

(The famous Libby Zion case in NYC involved a death due to combining meperidine and an MAOI)

Too much neuroleptic medication can cause what two problems, mainly?

1. Hypotension (mainly orthostatic)
2. Anticholinergic symptoms

What antiarrhythmic class should be avoided for patients taking neuroleptics, and also patients on digoxin or phenytoin?

Class 1a
(quinidine & procainamide)

**Patients taking neuroleptic medications are at risk for what idiosyncratic reaction?**

**Neuroleptic malignant syndrome (NMS)**

**What are the main features of neuroleptic malignant syndrome?**
(5 items – 3 are autonomic)

**Hyperthermia**
**Hypertension**
**Tachycardia**
**Muscle rigidity**
**Change of mental status**

How is serotonin syndrome (another toxidrome) different from NMS?
    (2 ways)

• No muscle rigidity
• Often mild, although can be serious

Is NMS dose related?

No

| How is NMS treated? | 1. <u>**Discontinue the neuroleptic!**</u> |
| | 2. **Supportive care** |
| | 3. **Alkalinize urine** – to protect kidneys if significant muscle breakdown is present |
| | 4. Paralysis if needed |
| | 5. Control temp |
| | |
| | (*Change* – Dantrolene, & other medications such as dopamine 2 (D2) receptor agonists, are still sometimes used, but evidence as to effectiveness is unclear) |
| **What is the toxicity of oral hypoglycemic agents?** | **Prolonged hypoglycemia (makes sense!)** |
| **How is oral hypoglycemic agent overdose treated, in general?** | **Glucose** **Glucagon (very short term)** **Admission or observation until drug is processed and no longer active** |
| **Which patient group is at greatest risk of severe hypoglycemia, with oral hypoglycemic ingestion/ overdose?** | **Young children (poor glycogen reserves)** |
| **In iron poisoning, how do you calculate the dose ingested?** | <u>**Elemental**</u> **iron/kg** |
| **How is iron ingestion treated?** | 1. **Whole-bowel irrigation** 2. **Chelation with deferoxamine** |
| How many phases are there to iron toxicity? | Four (same as Tylenol™, another common one) |
| What is the first phase of iron toxicity? | GI symptoms & sometimes shock! |
| What is the <u>last</u> phase of iron toxicity? | Scarring (of the gut) and recovery |
| After the first phase of GI symptoms, what happens in the second phase? | Quiescence (nothing – quiet phase) |

| | |
|---|---|
| Which iron toxicity phase features acidosis, liver injury, and sometimes coma? | The third (Between quiescence and scarring) |
| So, what are all four phases of the iron toxicity syndrome? | 1. GI & shock<br>2. Quiescent<br>3. Acidosis, liver injury, coma<br>4. Scarring & recovery (sometimes obstruction) |
| **Does charcoal bind iron?** | **No – iron is a metal** |
| What do the labs usually show in iron poisoning? | + anion gap<br>+ acidosis<br>↑ WBCs<br>↑ glucose |
| **Is an X-ray useful if iron ingestion is suspected?** | **Yes – it is radioopaque** |
| If you see the buzzword "vin rose" referring to urine, what are you supposed to think of? | Iron toxicity –<br>Urine that is "rosé wine colored" following deferoxamine (iron) chelation |
| How is lithium toxicity treated? | Supportive care<br><br>&<br><br>Hemodialysis if severe |
| The signs of lithium toxicity occur mainly in what two body systems? | CNS<br><br>&<br><br>Cardiac |
| What is the main problem lithium tends to create for the heart? | Long QT |
| What are the main CNS consequences of lithium overdose? | Seizure<br>Slurred speech<br>Coma |
| In what situation is a low serum level of lithium most likely to be toxic? | With chronic use |

Chronic lithium use results in toxicity at lower levels than acute ingestions do. Which is more life threatening, acute or chronic ingestions?

Acute ingestion
(25 % mortality vs. 9 % for chronic)

What electrolyte/fluid problems must you watch for, and correct, in lithium ingestions?

Hyponatremia

&

Dehydration

(both worsen toxicity)

**If the lithium ingestion seems to be mild, and the patient is not very symptomatic, what supportive care should be offered?**

1. **Hold lithium!**
2. **Lavage to remove tablets if reasonable**
3. **Maintain hydration & sodium level**
4. **Hold any diuretics (risk of dehydration)**

After an episode of lithium poisoning, what two systems may not recover completely?

CNS

&

Kidney

(lithium is renally excreted)

How useful is a lithium level to predicting toxicity in a lithium overdose?

Not great –
Response varies among individuals, and depending on acute vs. chronic ingestion (or both)

**Which metal is a common cause of acute poisoning deaths in children?**

**Iron**

**Which metal is a common cause of chronic poisoning in children?**

**Lead**

(acute ingestion is quite rare)

Which peripheral neuropathy is "classically" associated with lead poisoning?

Wrist drop

**What do you expect to see on the CBC of a patient with chronic lead poisoning?**

**Microcytic anemia**

**&**

**"Basophilic stippling" of the RBCs**

Tiny blue dots covering the surface of RBCs are called _____?

Basophilic stippling

Why might you want to get an abdominal X-ray on a lead toxicity patient?

If it's a child or pica patient, you might "see" the lead source in the gut (paint chips, etc.)

If a significant amount of lead were found on the KUB, what would you need to do?

Whole-bowel irrigation

(unlikely to happen – lead is rarely an acute ingestion)

**How is lead poisoning usually treated?**

**Chelation**

**Which chelation medications can be used for lead poisoning? (3)**

**BAL (British anti-Lewisite) DMSA EDTA**

**So, how does lead poisoning present?**

**Abdominal pain/anorexia Headache Learning/behavior problems**

Both lead & mercury cause problems by combining with sulfhydryl groups on molecules. Why does that binding cause a problem?

Enzyme activity is impeded

(Various enzymes are affected – most famously in heme synthesis, with lead poisoning)

**What oral cavity finding goes along with lead toxicity in children?**

**"Lead lines" in the gingiva**

(Dark lines where the gums meet the teeth – result of oral bacteria interacting with a high circulating lead level.)

At what lead level is lead poisoning automatically considered to be severe?

>50 mcg/dL

**If serum lead levels exceed 10 mcg/dL, what cognitive or behavioral effects are expected?**

**1. Short attention span 2. Cognitive decline 3. Antisocial behavior**

Lead can be chelated, but stores of lead in what body structure are difficult to remove?

Bone
(It is slowly released from bone)

| | |
|---|---|
| If the lead level begins to rise again after chelation, what is happening? | Bone is releasing it |
| If the lead level increases significantly after chelation, what should you do? | Chelate again |
| What dietary modifications are helpful for a lead poisoned child? | High calcium & iron diet<br><br>(They compete with lead in the gut) |
| After chelation, what should you expect with regard to the CNS changes associated with lead toxicity? | They are permanent |
| Are low levels of lead in the serum alright? | No –<br>Low levels still contribute to decreased cognitive functioning |
| What is the main problem to deal with in opiate overdose? | Respiratory depression/apnea |
| What are the other signs of opiate overdose? (other than respiratory depression) | Pinpoint pupils (usually)<br>Hypotension (mild)<br>CNS depression or coma |
| How can you reverse an opiate overdose? | Naloxone<br>(Narcan) |
| What must you be careful of, if you use naloxone?<br>(3) | 1. If you patient wakes up, s/he may vomit<br>2. Naloxone wears off long before the opiate does (& your patient might stop breathing if that happens!)<br>3. Chronic opioid users can be very angry and combative when woken and may have significant pain that is very hard to control |

| | |
|---|---|
| What is the long-acting form of naloxone called? (not widely used) | Naltrexone (Half-life = 72 h) |
| In addition to respiratory depression/apnea, what other problem sometimes develops with the lungs in opiate overdose? | Noncardiogenic pulmonary edema |
| What source of opiate is often "around the house" and available for accidental ingestion? | Lomotil™ (symptoms usually develop slowly) |
| **Rotatory nystagmus is a buzzword for what recreational drug ingestion or use?** | **PCP** **(+unusual strength)** |
| **A child presents with a history of intermittent abdominal pain. Routine CBC reveals anemia and RBCs with basophilic stippling. What is the likely diagnosis?** | **Lead toxicity** |
| **Patients using PCP are at risk for what kidney damaging problem?** | **Rhabdomyolysis** (probably due to over-exerting their muscles!) |
| If a PCP patient (and most other recreational drug users) has problems with hypertension after agitation has been controlled, what is your best choice to treat it? | Phentolamine or labetolol (or other meds with both alpha & beta-blocker effects) *(PCP can cause malignant hypertension, damaging end organs)* |
| How is PCP use handled medically? | Benzos & pentobarbital/propofol for the severely agitated |
| Do PCP users have problems with temperature regulation? | Sometimes – Hyperthermia |
| Other than insulin & oral hypoglycemics, which other substances often cause hypoglycemia? (4) | 1. ETOH (mainly in kids) 2. Salicylates OD 3. Phenytoin OD 4. Acetaminophen OD |

**If a patient presents with overdose and altered mental status, what must you always check?**

The *glucose*

**(Should check it for anyone with altered mental status – with or without OD)**

Poisoning from pesticides causes problems by what mechanism?

Too much acetylcholine – the breakdown enzyme is inhibited

**What is the name of the enzyme affected in organophosphate & carbamate insecticide poisoning?**

**Acetylcholinesterase**

**What is the main "toxidrome" you expect to see in pesticide poisoning?**

**Salivation
Lacrimation
Urination
Defecation
GI distress/emesis**

What toxidrome is expected with exposure to most nerve gases?

Also SLUDGE
(same mechanism)

**How are cholinergic toxidromes (those caused by too much ACh) treated?**

**Atropine
(It is a competitive inhibitor of ACh at muscarinic sites)**

With organophosphate pesticide toxicity, and nerve gases, what additional medication is needed for treatment?
(atropine + _____)

2-PAM

(aka pralidoxime)

What is the point of giving pralidoxime after certain cholinergic toxic exposures?

It prevents the permanent destruction of acetylcholinesterase

(without it, recovery depends on regeneration of the enzyme)

SLUDGE doesn't sound life-threatening, just annoying. Why is the cholinergic toxidrome potentially fatal?

2 reasons:

– The secretions are so copious they can interfere with breathing

– Constant ACh stimulation of respiratory and voluntary muscle results in paralysis

| | |
|---|---|
| What "class" of antiarrhythmic is quinidine? | Class 1a – sodium channel blockers<br><br>(Procainamide is also 1a) |
| What is the main danger of having too much quinidine? | Prolonged QT<br>&<br>Possible torsades |
| How can quinidine overdose be treated? | Isoproterenol<br>Pacing<br><br>(Magnesium for torsades, if needed) |
| **Ben-Gay® contains a high level of what toxin?** | **Oil of wintergreen<br>(a very toxic salicylate)** |
| **What is the odd pH presentation of salicylate overdose patients?** | **Initial respiratory alkalosis,<br>then metabolic acidosis** |
| How do children usually present, when they have ingested salicylates? | Hyperventilation<br>Diaphoresis &<br>Behavioral changes |
| In an acute salicylate poisoning, symptoms are usually most prominent in which system? | <u>Gut</u> distress |
| When a patient chronically taking salicylates becomes toxic, what types of symptoms are usually most noticeable? | CNS –<br>Tinnitus, seizures, coma, fever |
| Overall, a bad salicylate poisoning looks like a patient with what diagnosis _____? | Sepsis<br>(tachycardic, febrile, tachypneic, pulmonary edema, depressed LOC) |
| Why do salicylate patients hyperventilate? | Salicylates stimulate the CNS respiratory center |
| What is the underlying mechanism of salicylate toxicity (the way it produces the metabolic acidosis)? | "uncoupling of oxidative phosphorylation" (the cell can't use oxygen to make energy anymore) |

| | |
|---|---|
| What kind of metabolic acidosis does salicylate poisoning cause? (anion gap or non-anion gap) | Anion gap |
| **What pulmonary problem is sometimes seen in salicylate poisoning?** | **Pulmonary edema** |
| In addition to anion gap metabolic acidosis, what other metabolic derangements often occur with salicylate toxicity? | Hypoglycemia<br><br>&<br><br>Hypokalemia |
| For very severe cases of salicylate poisoning, what treatment will be needed? | Hemodialysis |
| Other than dialysis, how can salicylate overdose be treated? | Maintain glucose<br>Maintain potassium<br>Alkalinize (use bicarb) |
| What is the main goal of alkalinization in salicylate toxicity? | To trap salicylate ions in the urine<br><br>(The urine must have an alkaline pH or the treatment won't work.) |
| If you're giving bicarb, and the urine won't turn alkaline, what is the problem? | The potassium is low |
| Phenothiazine medications have many different effects. What effects do they have on the cardiovascular system? | Hypotension<br><br>&<br><br>Prolonged intervals (risk of torsades) |
| The CNS effects of phenothiazines, (sedation, psychosis, and seizures), along with heat stroke and urinary retention effects, are due to the _____ & _____ effects of phenothiazines? | Anticholinergic<br><br>&<br><br>Antihistamine |

| | |
|---|---|
| **What reaction to phenothiazines is commonly seen and easily treated?** | **Dystonic reaction**<br><br>**(can also occasionally occur with PCP & ketamine)** |
| **What is a dystonic reaction? (3)** | **Torticollis**<br>**Eye deviation**<br>**Facial grimacing** |
| **What bad complication can (rarely) occur in a dystonic reaction?** | **Laryngospasm** |
| **How are dystonic reactions treated?** | **Benadryl®**<br>**(Diphenhydramine)** |
| Why can rapid infusion of (regular) phenytoin be life-threatening? | Can cause cardiovascular collapse |
| Why can phenytoin infusion cause cardiovascular collapse, but fosphenytoin will not? | It was the polypropylene glycol vehicle in the Dilantin®/Phenytoin that caused the problem –<br>Fosphenytoin doesn't have it! |
| Is an oral ingestion of phenytoin likely to be life-threatening, if it is large? | No –<br>Although it can cause coma |
| **How can (oral) Dilantin®/ phenytoin overdose be treated?** | **Single-dose activated charcoal**<br>(multi-dose sometimes used in adults & older adolescents – efficacy unclear)<br><br>**(Dialysis is traditionally not used** – recent literature suggests that it may have a moderate helpful effect, but this is controversial) |
| **What are the symptoms of phenytoin toxicity?** | **CNS problems, usually –**<br>**Ataxia**<br>**Slurred speech**<br>**Nystagmus**<br>**Vomiting** |
| Can phenytoin have cardiac effects? | Yes – it affects sodium channels |

What should you watch for in terms of cardiovascular effects of excess phenytoin?

Bradycardia

&

*QRS widening*

How should a levetiracetam (Keppra®) overdose be treated? (3)

Activated charcoal (single dose)

Supportive care

Hemodialysis is an option for severe overdose (generally not required)

What two drugs in the xanthine class are overdose problems?

Caffeine

&

Theophylline

**What are the symptoms of excess xanthines?**

**Tachycardia**
**Vomiting**
**Seizures**

**(Bad day at the Starbucks®!)**

**How does theophylline overdose happen?**

**Accidental ingestion**

&

*Drug interaction!!*
**(It is protein bound, and the level suddenly goes up if it is pushed off the protein.)**

As with most other chronically used medications, greater toxicity is seen at lower levels when theophylline use is _____? (chronic or acute)

Chronic

In xanthine overdose, how well does the drug level correspond to toxicity?

Well in acute overdose,
Poor in chronic

What electrolyte abnormality can occur with xanthine toxicity?

Hypokalemia

| | |
|---|---|
| **Other than coffee, tea, & soda, where are your patients likely to encounter caffeine (in sufficient quantities to overdose)?**<br>(3) | Diet pills<br><br>**Over-the-counter stimulants (like "No Doze®")**<br><br>**"Energy" drinks!** |
| **Which commonly encountered medications are likely to "bump" the theophylline level up?**<br>(3) | **Erythromycin**<br>**Cimetidine**<br>**Ciprofloxacin** |
| Due to the hepatic processing of the drug, certain medical conditions also increase theophylline levels – such as? | Liver failure<br>&<br>CHF |
| In addition to low potassium, what other electrolyte changes are seen with xanthine overdose? | Low Magnesium<br>&<br>Low Phosphorous |
| **Do xanthines have cardiac effects other than tachycardia?** | **Yes –**<br>**SVT is fairly common** |
| **If supportive care is not enough, how do you treat a xanthine overdose?**<br>(2 meds & 2 ion related) | **β-blockers (cardiac effect)**<br>**Phenobarb (for seizures)**<br>**Mg repletion**<br>**Manage electrolytes** |
| **The main symptoms of tricyclic antidepressant overdose come from their _____ & _____ effects.** | **Antihistamine**<br>&<br>**Anticholinergic** |
| **What symptoms are noticeable early on in TCA overdose?**<br>(5) | 1. **Tachycardia**<br>2. **Dilated pupils**<br>3. *Warm, dry, & slightly flushed skin*<br>4. **Ileus**<br>5. **Sedation**<br><br>**(skin findings often featured in vignettes)** |
| **What unusual pattern of blood pressure findings is seen in TCA overdose?** | **Hypertension,**<br>**followed by hypotension** |

| | |
|---|---|
| Why do TCAs cause the unusual pattern of hypertension followed by hypotension? | Catecholamine reuptake is blocked → initial hypertension<br><br>Then,<br><br>Alpha blockade produces hypotension |
| **How well does the TCA level correlate to the findings in overdose?** | **Not well** |
| **What is the main concern with regard to cardiac effects of TCAs?** | **QRS widening** |
| **TCAs act like what class of cardiac rhythm drugs?** | **1a**<br><br>**(Sodium channel blockers like quinidine & procainamide)** |
| In general, the cardiac effects of TCAs fall into what general categories?<br>   (3) | 1. Interval prolongation<br>2. QRS widening<br>3. Right axis finding (e.g. right axis deviation or RBBB) |
| **What is the mainstay of treatment for TCA overdose?** | **Bicarb!!!**<br>**(titrate to width of QRS)** |
| How is the hypotension of TCA overdose treated? | Bicarb, hydration, & alpha agonists (e.g. norepinephrine) |
| Is multidose charcoal useful for TCA overdose? | Yes |
| Why does bicarb treat the cardiac toxicity of TCA overdose?<br>   (3 possibilities) | Several effects –<br>Correction of acidic pH improves heart contractility<br><br>Traditionally taught that TCA binds to proteins more in an alkaline environment (removing it from the heart) – this may or may not be the case<br><br>Sodium load may help to overwhelm the sodium channels, partly correcting sodium channel function |

| | |
|---|---|
| **How are seizures due to TCA overdose treated?** | **Benzos** <br> & <br> **Phenobarb** <br> (Propofol has also been used) |
| Which TCAs are most likely to cause seizure? | Maprotiline <br> & <br> Amoxapine |
| **Does sodium bicarb treat TCA-induced seizures?** | **No!!!** <br> **Use benzos, if seizures are prolonged or frequent** |
| **In addition to lack of efficacy, why else might you want to avoid giving phenytoin for TCA overdose seizures?** | **It could worsen arrhythmia –** <br><br> **Its sodium channel activity is similar to the TCAs** |
| If seizure occurs with TCA overdose, when do you typically see it? | First 6–8 h post-ingestion <br><br> (most likely in first 3 h) |
| **Which antiarrhythmic classes of medication must be avoided in a TCA overdose patient with dysrhythmia?** <br> **(3)** | 1. **β-blockers** <br> 2. **Calcium channel blockers** <br> 3. **Sodium channel blockers** <br> 4. **Class III agents (amiodarone, bretylium, sotalol)** <br><br> (β-blkrs & calcium channel blkrs contribute to hypotension – <br> Class III agents may further lengthen the QT interval, increasing chances for a malignant arrhythmia) |
| How can you treat TCA arrhythmia that does not respond to bicarb? | Lidocaine and/or magnesium sulfate <br><br> Or <br><br> Synchronized cardioversion or pacing |

**Hypotension with TCA overdose should be treated with fluids and bicarb before pressors are given. If a pressor is needed, which one is best?**

**Norepinephrine or phenylephrine (they directly compete with the TCA at α sites)**

Which pressor should be avoided in TCA overdose, and why?

Dopamine –
Often causes vasodilation in this setting

(partly relies on endogenous catecholamine release for its effect – those catecholamines may already be depleted)

How could a patient become slowly cyanide toxic in the hospital?

Remained on nitroprusside too long

(breakdown product is cyanide – toxicity develops slowly)

**If an important vital sign is missing from a toxicology vignette on the boards, what should you assume?**

**It is a clue –
The missing vital sign is important to the toxidrome**

In the past, Diamox (carbonic anhydrase inhibitor) has sometimes been suggested as a way to alkalinize your patient. Why is it no longer recommended?

It produces metabolic acidosis over time

**Especially in pediatrics, what fluid issue must you be aware of when alkalinizing your patient?**

**Fluid overload**

Some important toxins that respond well to alkalinization are _____?
  (3)

1. TCAs
2. Phenobarb
3. Salicylates

**For chelation therapy of iron overdose, how is deferoxamine given?**

**IV
(PO cannot be used)**

What are the main consequences of mercury exposure for fetuses?
  (4)

Blindness
Deafness
Seizures
Microcephaly

| | |
|---|---|
| Methyl mercury ingestion (from fish) presents with what neurological findings? | Ataxia<br>Paresthesias<br>Tremors<br>Dysarthria<br>Special senses changes |
| If methyl mercury ingestion progresses, what is its usual course? | Dementia<br>&<br>Death |
| How is mercury poisoning treated? | BAL<br>(British anti-Lewisite, also known as dimercaprol) |
| **A family who has been traveling together by car on a long-distance trip present with flu-like symptoms. They usually feel fine when they wake up, but develop symptoms during the day. What toxin exposure should you think of?** | **Carbon monoxide** |
| What is the main effect of levetiracetam overdose (Keppra®)? | CNS depression & potentially coma |
| What is the mainstay of treatment for a levetiracetam overdose? | Supportive care – hemodialysis can be used but is generally not needed |
| In a young child, refusal to drink or copious salivation could indicate what toxic exposure? | Corrosive ingestion (acid or alkali) |
| Where do kids typically find acids to drink? | Toilet bowl cleaners |
| Where do kids typically find alkalis to drink? | Drain cleaners |
| **How well can you judge the condition of the esophagus, based on oral & perioral burns?** | **Not well** |

**Iron ingestions are famous**          **Pyloric stenosis**
**for leading to gut scarring and**
**obstruction. What sort of gastric**
**obstruction is especially common**
**in these patients?**

**If a patient presents more than**      **Give *N*-acetylcysteine while waiting**
**four hours after a concerning**        **for the initial level**
**acetaminophen ingestion, what**
**should you do for initial**
**management?**

**What kind of toxin is Jimsonweed?**    **Anticholinergic**

# Chapter 5
# General Prevention Question and Answer Items

| | |
|---|---|
| **All states screen newborns for which two disorders?** | **PKU & hypothyroidism** |
| Most states also screen for what endocrine disorder? | Congenital adrenal hyperplasia |
| What other classes of disorders are typically screened for? | Hemoglobinopathies |
| | Fatty acid oxidation disorders |
| | Organic acid disorders |
| | Amino acid disorders |
| Many states are also beginning to screen for which immune disorders? | SCID disorders |
| | (Severe Combined ImmunoDeficiency – allowing diagnosis before the child becomes ill, hopefully) |
| The PKU screen is the most complicated of the newborn tests. What are the special rules for the timing of the test? | If the test is done at <24 h old, must be repeated between 1 and 2 weeks of age |
| | (the metabolite might not have built up in 24 h) |
| What procedures can cause PKU screening to be inaccurate? | Blood transfusions & dialysis |
| What procedures can cause hemoglobinopathy screening to be inaccurate? | Transfusion |
| | (After all, it's not *their* hemoglobin you're testing, if they've been transfused!) |

© Springer Science+Business Media New York 2015
C.M. Houser, *Pediatric Tricky Topics, Volume 1*,
DOI 10.1007/978-1-4939-1859-1_5

**What is the rule for ophthalmology referral depending on the difference in acuity between the two eyes?**

**If there is more than one line discrepancy in what the R vs. L eye can read – Refer!**

(there are also specific acuity requirements that vary by age – please refer to the ophthalmology section in Tricky Topics II)

At what age should you test kids for strabismus with the "cover/ uncover" test?

Toddler – preschool

Between ages 3 and 5, it is difficult for kids to use a standard eye chart. What test can be used instead?

The random-dot-E test (E's in different orientations)

How often should school-aged children and adolescents have their vision checked?

Annually

By 4 months old, what sorts of visual behavior can you check to assess vision?

Conjugate gaze
Object tracking

(red reflex should also be present, of course)

In young children, hearing can be tested with evoked potentials (ABR or BAER testing).
What newer, simpler, modality for testing young children is now available?

Evoked-oto-acoustic-emissions (EOAE)

(easier to use, but more false positives)

How often does the AAP recommend formal hearing testing?

Earliest formal hearing testing possible is age 3 –
Test in preschool,
Kindergarten,
Grades 1, 3, 5, & either 7 or 9 in the US educational system

(approximately ages 3, 5, 6, 8, 10, & 12–14 years)

*(and screening at birth, of course!)*

**Which kids need a hearing screening, based on their particular history?**
  **(3)**

1. **Parental concern about language development**
2. **history of infection that might cause hearing loss**
3. **history of ototoxic meds**

(sometimes also needed for head trauma or neurodegenerative diseases)

By what age should all infants have an initial hearing screening, and how should that screening be done?

By 1 month old!

Physiological testing
(not just clinical impression)

If the initial hearing screening is abnormal or can't be interpreted, what should be done?

Rescreen the infant promptly – if it remains abnormal, then referral for medical & audiological exam is required

The AAP has set a standard for all congenitally deaf children to be identified by what age?

3 months

**What is the main reason to screen for hearing loss?**

**Big effect on speech/language development**

**Is universal screening for elevated cholesterol in children recommended?**

**Yes –**
**One time between ages 9 and 11 years**

**Repeat between ages 17 and 21 years**

*(This is a change from prior recommendations!)*

**Which children in the other age groups (2–8 year olds & 12–16 year olds) should also have lipid screening?**

  **(4 groups –**
**1 parental factor**
**1 behavioral factor**
**1 family history factor**
**1 set of patient medical factors)**

**Parent with dyslipidemia or total cholesterol >240**

**Child who smokes**

**Child with DM, HTN, lipid-related medical condition (moderate to high risk), or BMI $\geq$95 %**

**Family history positive for early atherosclerotic disease**

What qualifies as "family history of early atherosclerotic disease?"

MI, stroke, angina, coronary artery bypass graft/stent/or angioplasty, or sudden cardiac death at <55 years old in a male relative, or <65 years old in a female relative

| | |
|---|---|
| Which relatives "count" for the positive family history of cardiovascular disease? | Parent, grandparent, *aunt/uncle*, or sibling |
| What are considered high or moderate risk factor lipid-related conditions? | HTN<br>Cigarette smoker<br>HDL <40<br>DM |
| Which additional medical disorders are high or moderate risk factors for lipid-related conditions?<br>(5) | Heart or kidney transplant<br><br>Kidney disease, including nephrotic syndrome<br><br>HIV infection<br><br>Kawasaki's disease with presence, or history of, aneurysms<br><br>Chronic inflammatory (rheumatological) disorders |
| Children must usually be at least how old to qualify for lipid lowering medication treatment? | 10 years old |
| At what confirmed LDL level should a child generally be started on statin therapy? | ≥190 mg/dL<br><br>(10 years old or older) |
| Patients with confirmed LDL levels ≥130, but less than 190 mg/dL, should be started on a statin if what other conditions are met?<br>(2) | Clinical coronary vascular disease is present<br><br>OR<br><br>At least three risk factors are present (at least one high risk & two moderate risk, depending on the LDL level)<br><br>(& *10 years old or older*) |
| Why is lipid screening avoided in children ages 12–16 years old, if possible? | High false negative & low sensitivity & specificity in this age group, when you try to correlate the current result to adult lipid (LDL) levels |
| Which lipid test should you order, for screening purposes? | The fasting lipid profile |

| | |
|---|---|
| At what triglyceride level should you automatically refer to a specialist? | ≥500 mg/dL |
| At what LDL level should you automatically refer to a specialist? | ≥250 mg/dL |
| Should abnormal fasting lipid profile results be repeated? If so, when? | Yes, repeat at least one time<br><br>Wait for at least 2 weeks between measures (but not more than 3 months!) |
| At what triglyceride (TG) level might a child need to be started on a TG lowering medication? | ≥200<br><br>Consider omega-3 fish oil therapy, also |
| **At what age should you start screening children's BP, and how often should you recheck it?** | **3 years –**<br>**Recheck annually** |
| **If you think a child's blood pressure is abnormal, what will you need to do to confirm it?** | **Same as an adult – take three readings on three different days**<br>**(they should all be abnormal if it's real)**<br><br>*If the BP is from a machine (oscillometry) it must be confirmed with BP by auscultation!* |
| There are three types of elevated BP. What are they?<br><br>*(Note: These categories have been updated in the last few years!)* | Prehypertension<br>(91–95 % for age)<br><br>Stage 1 hypertension<br>(>95 % for age but <99 %+5 mmHg)<br><br>Stage 2 hypertension<br>(≥99 %+5 mmHg) |
| **If a child is identified with prehypertension, what should you do?** | **Evaluate need for weight management, educate on activity, & check CV risk factors**<br><br>&<br><br>**Repeat BP check in 6 months** |

Which interventions should ALL children identified with prehypertension or hypertension receive?
(4)

Weight management evaluation

BP follow-up checks

Activity counseling

Diet guidance

If a child is identified with Stage 1 hypertension (HTN), what needs to be done & how often should they be rechecked?

Basic HTN work-up

&

Recheck BP in 3–6 months

What is considered the "basic work-up" for a child with some degree of HTN, according to current guidelines?

History & physical exam (including family history & sleep history)

CBC, renal panel, lipids, glucose, & urinalysis

Renal & cardiac ultrasound

Should any of these children be started on antihypertensive medications?

Yes –
Those with LVH (left ventricular hypertrophy) or secondary HTN should be started on medication immediately (+treat underlying cause, if secondary)

+

Patients whose pressure remains Stage 1 after 3–6 months of follow-up

If a child is identified with stage 2 hypertension, what needs to be done?

Refer to a pediatric HTN expert within 1 week

OR

Begin treatment & work-up immediately

At what age should fasting glucose first be tested?

Approximately age 10 years, or at the beginning of puberty (if it is before 10 years)

Children over 2 years old can be considered for testing, depending on clinical concern & risk factors.

**Which kids should have a fasting glucose screening test?**

**Overweight + two risk factors from the categories:**

**Family history**
**Race/ethnicity &**
**Signs of insulin resistance**

**Which family history risk factors are used to screen children in need of a fasting blood glucose measurement?**

**History of type 2 diabetes in a 1st- or 2nd-degree relative**

**Within the USA, which races or ethnic groups are considered to be at increased risk for type 2 diabetes?**

**Native American**
**Pacific Islander**
**African American**
**Hispanic American**
**Asian American**

**Which signs of insulin resistance are used to determine the need to screen for DM in children?**

**Acanthosis nigricans (skin finding)**

**Hypertension or lipid disorder**

**Polycystic ovary syndrome (PCOS)**

How is overweight defined, in the American Diabetic Association's (ADA) guidelines for which children require fasting glucose screening?
   (3 ways)

BMI >85th % for age & sex

Weight >120 % for height

Weight for height >85th %

If initial fast blood glucose test results are not suspicious for DM, how often should the child be rescreened?

Every 2 years

What qualifies as "family history of early atherosclerotic disease?"

MI, stroke, angina, coronary artery bypass graft/stent/or angioplasty, or sudden cardiac death at <55 years old in a male, or <65 years old in a female relative

Which relatives "count" for positive family history of cardiovascular disease?

Parent, grandparent, aunt/uncle, or sibling

| | |
|---|---|
| **If you need to do a lipid screen, what is the right test to order?** | **"Fasting serum lipid profile" (total cholesterol, HDL, LDL, & triglycerides)** |
| What is the recommended diet for children in the first year of life, to reduce risks of future cardiovascular disease? | Breastfeeding only (if possible), with gradual introduction of solids |
| After age 12 months, what sort of milk is recommended? | 2 % or fat-free milk |
| If a DASH-type diet is recommended for your patient, what does that mean, and why (mainly) is it recommended? | Diet high in fruit & vegetables, nuts, whole grains, & low-fat or fat-free milk products (sugar content is low)<br><br>• It is thought to promote cardiovascular health |
| What is the main beverage recommended to foster cardiovascular health, for children between the ages of 2 and 21 years old? | Fat-free unflavored milk (& encourage water) |
| What is the maximum time per day children older than 1 year old should be viewing a screen? (television, computer, etc.) | Maximum is 1–2 hours – *Even if it is high quality programming*<br><br>Less is preferred! |
| As children become adolescents, is it a good idea to allow them more freedom & privacy, by having a television or other screens, in their own room? | NO – Not recommended from a health perspective |
| For children between the ages of 5 and 21 years old, how often should they have moderate-to-vigorous exercise? | Daily! |
| Why is venous blood sampling for lead level better than capillary sticks? | Finger stick (capillary stick) can be contaminated with lead on the skin |

If a child lives in an historic home, or historic community, is he/she likely to need a lead level?

Yes
(home built before 1950, or area with >27 % of homes built before 1950)

Which kids may need lead screening (what age group)?

6 months to 6 years

**At what lead level is treatment required?**

**>10 μg/dL**
(although recent studies have shown decline in cognitive performance at levels even lower than 10)

One risk factor for lead toxicity has to do with parental activities. What is it?

Job or hobby with caretaker exposure to lead (they take it home on clothing/skin)

In a non-abusive household situation, is it possible to find parents feeding their children lead?

Yes – lead is often found in folk medicines, particularly those produced in developing countries, and also in ceramic pottery and pans used to prepare meals

At what age is it recommended that pediatricians ask children about their personal history of tobacco use?

5–10 years old

At what age are pediatricians recommended to speak with children about the bad consequences of tobacco use?

5–10 years old

**Does the AAP recommend screening Hgb/Hct universally?**

**Yes – between 9 and 12 months OR AT ANY TIME if risk factors for iron deficiency are present**

What are the main risk factors for iron deficiency in infants?

Prematurity or low birth weight

Exclusively breastfed without iron supplementation beyond 4 months old

Lead exposure

Weaning to diet low in iron

Which ethnicity is known to be at increased risk for low iron states?

Those of Mexican American descent

Should children with other chronic health conditions be considered at risk for iron deficiency?

Yes, both children with poor growth & those with chronic health conditions may have increased nutritional needs, or altered nutrition due to their condition

Why is iron deficiency important?

Big impact –
Cognitive impact occurs before iron deficiency anemia can be detected

**Which adolescents should have a screening H/H?**

**Athletes**

&

**menstruating females (annually)**

If you are going to screen children for abnormal H/H, when must you avoid drawing the blood?

During, or for a few weeks after, an acute illness
(because transient anemia is common then)

AAP recommends annual urine dipsticks for which patient population?

Sexually active adolescent males and females

**Does AAP recommend a universal urinalysis screening?**

**No**

*(Note: This is a change from previous recommendations!)*

**Is universal screening for TB recommended by the AAP?**

**No**

Is it alright to use the "multipuncture" test to evaluate for TB?

No – that is another way of saying "tuberculin tine test," and we are not allowed to use that one

**If you don't know a child's history well enough to evaluate risk factors for exposure to TB, what is the recommended approach to TB prevention?**

**Use the validated "TB Risk-Assessment Questionnaire" with either the parent or the adolescent patient**

*Any positive response means that the Mantoux test for TB response should be placed*

| | |
|---|---|
| Is it alright to place a PPD on a patient who has previously received the BCG immunization? | Yes |
| How do you read a PPD on a patient who was immunized with the BCG? | Same as other patients |
| **What determines whether the PPD is positive or negative?** | **Amount of induration in millimeters** |
| **How long do you have to wait, after placing the PPD, to read it?** | **48–72 h** (not longer, not shorter, just right – like Goldilocks) |
| **Although some patient groups are considered positive with smaller amounts of induration, how much induration is needed for patient's with no risk factors to be positive on the PPD?** | **15 mm** |
| On the boards, is it a good idea to do parental counseling at each visit? | Yes – but choose the topics depending on the child's age and reason for visit |
| When little babies come in for pedi visits, what skin care issue should you be sure to talk about? | Sun protection – meaning keeping the baby out of the sun! Very vulnerable skin (Infants older than 6 months may be protected with sunscreen, but exposure avoidance remains important.) |
| For very young babies, what advice should you give regarding "spoiling" the child with too much attention/cuddling? | Not possible! |
| Is it the pediatrician's place to ask parents what arrangements they have made for childcare? | Yes |
| Before children can ambulate, what is the major drowning risk that you must discuss with parents? | Baths – (counsel about supervision, amount of water, securing infant) |

| | |
|---|---|
| At what age should you begin routinely counseling about drugs and sex? | Age 10 |
| At what age should you refer your patients for their first dental exam? | 12 months |
| **When should you recommend that your patients use protective helmets?** | **Any activity with increased velocity – bike riding, roller blading, etc.** |
| **You should routinely check whether your patients' families are using what essential protective device when in vehicles?** | **Car seats/booster seats/seat belts** |
| **You need to counsel parents to place the car seat in what orientation for very young children?** | **Backwards** |
| **When should the car seat face forward?** | **As late as possible – the current recommendation is after the child is 2 years old** |
| **A child should be a minimum of how big before the car seat is changed to the forward position?** | **2 years old – there is no weight recommendation anymore!** *(This is a change! It used to be that 20 pounds was the limit for facing the rear.)* |
| Is it alright for children to be restrained by lap belts *only,* if they are riding in the back seat? | No – risk of internal (GI) organ perforation and Chance fracture of the vertebra with impact |
| **When is it alright for children to ride in the front passenger seat?** | **When they are taller than 5 feet and at least 13 years old, unless the airbag is disabled** |
| Ideally, where should small children be seated in a vehicle? | Back seat, central area (away from the vehicle frame) |
| **What vitamin supplement should you recommend for all exclusively breastfed infants?** | **Vitamin D** |

Recommendations regarding the absolute quantity of daily vitamin D to recommend to children & adults vary. Which children, though, are likely to be at special risk for vitamin D deficiency, if not supplemented?

(4 groups)

Those in Northern climates

Darker skinned

Those with little sun exposure

Those with gut conditions rendering absorption difficult (e.g., IBD or gastric bypass patients)

How is the infant sleep pattern for REM sleep different from that of adults?

>50 % of infant sleep time is REM – adults have much less

Why is increased REM sleep sometimes a problem in establishing good sleeping habits in small infants?

Parents sometimes misinterpret the REM sleep as awakening, and complain that the baby isn't "sleeping through the night"

(it becomes a problem if the parent is picking the child up during those times)

In what age range will infants usually nap twice each day?

12–18 months

What is the usual nap pattern after about 18 months of age?

One nap per day until age 4 years

(75 % of children give up their nap by age 5)

Toddlers are most likely to tolerate going to bed when parents do what?

Establish and follow a routine

On average, how much time per day does a 2-week-old baby spend crying?

About 2 hours

What is the pattern for amount of crying in the first 3 months of life?

Starts around 2 hours per day
Goes to 3 hours at 6 weeks
Drops to 2 hours at 3 months

**Is corporal punishment, as long as it does not result in injury or marks on the skin, an acceptable means of discipline on the boards?**

**No – not at all**

**What is the best way to advise parents to discipline young children – <age 5 years?**

**Time-outs – 1 min for each year of life**

| | |
|---|---|
| If a child leaves a time-out the parent has assigned, what is the parent supposed to do? | 1. Tell child to go back to time out<br>2. If child won't go back voluntarily, escort the child back |
| What is a key to success with the time-out method? | Limit interaction with the child while in time-out (as close to no interaction as possible) |
| **What does the AAP recommend for disciplining children older than age 5?** | **Loss of privileges** |
| **If corporal punishment is an answer choice on the boards, should you ever choose it?** | **NO!** |
| **What advice are you supposed to give for families that choose to keep firearms in the home?** | • **Lock the firearm up**<br>• **Keep ammunition in a separate, locked location** |
| **Should you routinely ask families about whether they keep firearms in the home?** | **Yes!** |
| **After children become ambulatory, what drowning risks should you be sure to discuss?** | **Pools (both private home & public pools), natural bodies of water, bath tubs, and "wash buckets" like the ones people use for washing cars & doing cleaning** |
| Do swimming lessons decrease a child's risk for drowning? | No.<br><br>(Studies show this – I know it's hard to believe!) |
| **What household appliance issues should you counsel your families about?**<br>**(5)** | • **Hot water heater – no more than 120°**<br>• **Smoke detectors**<br>• **Carbon monoxide detectors(**<br>• **Stove tops (all pan handles turned IN & flame/burn issues)**<br>• **Irons for clothing** |
| **Why do toys often have that warning – "Not intended for children <3 years of age?"** | **Small parts – choking hazard – families need to be counseled about choking hazards**<br><br>(It's not about whether the child is "advanced" for his age!!!) |

| | |
|---|---|
| **What poisoning risks do families often forget about?** | • **Plants inside & outside the home (stop sucking on that foxglove!)**<br>• **Meds belonging to other family members**<br><br>**(Naturally cleaners and detergents below the sink or in other accessible areas including garages should be removed before ambulatory children are in the house!)** |
| If your patient is honored to make the varsity team, but is considerably smaller than the size of the other boys/girls, what should you counsel? | Special protection, or deferring play on the varsity team, might be indicated to prevent injury<br><br>(age- and size-matched teams are generally preferred) |
| **Is it fine for your patients to play soccer without shin guards, etc.?** | **No – all safety gear appropriate to the sport should be worn** |
| **What do you need to tell young kids and their families about meeting new animals?** | **Bite prevention – don't approach animals you don't know, animals that are eating, animals with young, don't startle animals, etc.** |
| **What is the most effective drowning prevention tool for children?** | Fenced pools –<br>Meaning the pool, itself, is fenced – not the entire backyard, which still leaves the household children at risk |
| **Infants & young toddlers should avoid what unfortunately shaped foods?** | **Things shaped like the airway – especially if they're firm<br>(For example: grapes, peanuts, hard candy)** |
| **Is it alright to give infants/toddlers popcorn, if they are old enough to be eating corn products?** | **No – still an aspiration risk** |
| **What's wrong with feeding toddlers hotdogs?** | **<u>Whole</u> or <u>sliced</u> hotdogs can occlude the airway** |
| **Raw fruit and vegetables are good for people, in general. Are they good for toddlers?** | **Yes, if they are cut up – large pieces are an aspiration risk** |

# Chapter 6
# General Research and Statistics Question and Answer Items

Sensitivity tells you how good the test is for finding _____ ?

Positives

(people with the disease, people who respond, etc.)

How do you calculate sensitivity? (no panic allowed!)

$$\frac{\textbf{True positives found}}{\textbf{All true}\left(\textbf{real}\right)\textbf{positives}}$$

(True positives with positive results ÷ The total number of positives that *should* have been found)

Specificity tells you how good a test is for finding _____ ?

Negatives –
**Correctly ruling out the negatives**

(people without disease, people who don't respond, etc.)

How do you calculate specificity?

$$\frac{\textbf{True negatives found}}{\textbf{All true}\left(\textbf{real}\right)\textbf{negatives}}$$

(True negatives with a negative result ÷ The total number of negatives that *should* have been found)

What does "prevalence" mean?

**The fraction of the population that has whatever you are looking for**

(For example, if 5 of 100 people in the population have DM, then the prevalence is 5/100 or 0.05)

© Springer Science+Business Media New York 2015
C.M. Houser, *Pediatric Tricky Topics, Volume 1*,
DOI 10.1007/978-1-4939-1859-1_6

**Do sensitivity and specificity change, depending on the prevalence of a disease?**

**NO**
**(they are prevalence *independent*)**

Note:
The "predictive value" tests will change with prevalence

**A popular test item asks what will happen when you move a screening test's threshold up or down. If you raise a test's threshold, so that it is *harder* to get a positive result, what is the effect on the sensitivity?**

(For example, if you were using 100 as the cutoff for a normal glucose, and you increase that to 120, will you find more, or fewer, diabetics?)

**It's decreased**

**You will find fewer diabetics**
(missing more true positives)

**What if you move your test's threshold so that it is *easier* to get a positive result? What will happen to sensitivity then?**

(For example, if you change your glucose threshold from 120 to 105 for a diagnosis of possible DM . . .)

**Sensitivity will be great!**
*(You will find nearly all true positives!)*

Mnemonic:
Remember sensitivity by thinking of someone with "sensitive skin." If you send them into the woods to test for poison ivy, and it's there – they'll find it for you! If you send a non-responder (low-sensitivity skin), you'll never know it was there.

**When you move a test's threshold so that it's harder to get a positive result (e.g., a glucose of 200 to qualify for DM, instead of 120) what does that do to specificity for the test?**

**Better specificity –**
**When you say the patient has DM, you'll almost always be right!**

Mnemonic:
Think of "specificity" as a high anxiety kind of a gal. She doesn't want to make a mistake, so she's reluctant to answer unless she's *certain* she's right. When specificity is high, almost everyone selected will be a true positive (but a bunch of true positives are often missed!)

**What effect does it have on specificity, if you move your test's threshold, so that it is easier to get a positive result?**

Specificity is lower –
You're now identifying lots of people who *don't* have the disease, in addition to those who do.

**Does the positive predictive value (PPV) statistic depend on the prevalence of a disease?**

Yes

**Positive predictive value is classically used in what setting?**

*(popular test item)*

To decide whether something should be used as a screening test

**In words, what does the "positive predictive value" tell you?**

How valuable, or useful, it is to you as a clinician, if you get a positive result for a patient

If the test's positive predictive value is high, then the clinician can feel confident that a positive result means the patient really *is* positive, in nearly every case.

**How do you calculate the positive predictive value of a test?**

$$\frac{\text{True positives it found}}{\text{All persons labeled pos}}$$

(True positives with positive results ÷ Total number of positive results)

**What about negative predictive value – what does that mean, in regular words?**

It is how confident you can be that a negative result is a true negative

**How do you calculate the negative predictive value of a test?**

$$\frac{\text{True negatives it found}}{\text{All persons labeled neg}}$$

(True negatives with negative results ÷ Total number of negative results)

**If you have to calculate something on the exam, what size of population should you assume if that information is not given?**

1 million or 100,000 usually make for the easiest calculations

**Odds ratio – How on earth can I remember how to calculate the odds ratio?**

**Step 1 – Make a $2 \times 2$ table for whatever is being compared. Don't worry about which label you put where.**

**Step 2 – Identify the cells that match (+result & +disease, for example), and the cells that are mixed (+result & no disease, for example)**

**Step 3 – Multiply the ones that match over the ones that are mixed**

**What does the odds ratio formula look like, without the steps?**

$$\frac{(+,\,+)\quad(-,\,-)}{(+,\,-)\quad(-,+)}$$

$$\text{Multiply}: \frac{\text{matching}}{\text{mixed}}$$

**If you raise a test's threshold, what happens to the specificity?**

**It's improved**

**There are fewer false positives**

**What is a 95 % confidence interval?**

**The range of values in which the true value will be found – in 95 % of cases**

**As an example, if we measured the height of men from Norway, and found that the average height in our sample was 6 feet 2 in., and the heights of our subjects were pretty similar (little variation), a sample 95 % confidence might be . . .?**

**Mean of 6 feet 2 in. with a 95 % confidence interval of +/− 2 in.**

(The true value, with 95 % confidence, lies somewhere between 6 feet and 6 feet 4 in.)

**If a confidence interval is given for a statistic that can work out to zero, then how can you tell whether it is statistically significance?**

**(For example, a risk difference statistic)**

**If the confidence interval includes zero (often referred to as "crossing zero"), then the result is *not significant* – (because zero would mean no difference)**

*If it does not cross zero, it is significant*

**If a confidence interval is given for a statistic that can work out to one, how can you tell whether it is a statistically significant result? (For example, an odds ratio or relative risk)**

**If the confidence interval includes 1.0, then the result is *not significant* – (because one would mean no difference)**

*If it does not cross one, it is significant*

Standard deviations & standard error are not reported very much in current medical literature. They are still in the curriculum for pediatrics, though. In general terms, what is a "standard error" & with what kind of data could you use it?

Standard error measures how much variation is in the data collected

It is used for regular number data (things like height)

(Example: If you were studying height, and in your sample you had people who were very short through very tall, then the standard error would be large.)

What is standard deviation, then?

It tells you, in numerical form (in numbers), how close to the mean most of the studied population lies

(standard error is used in calculating the standard deviation, so they are closely related)

So if the standard deviation is very small, is that good?

Usually, yes –
It shows that results were consistent & near to a central value

What sort of study often uses the "relative risk statistic?"

Those looking at exposure to something, usually as a risk factor for disease development

In words, how is relative risk calculated?
(it actually makes sense)
Officially, how would you write out the calculation for relative risk?

$$\frac{\text{Proportion positive with exposure}}{\text{Proportion positive without exposure}}$$

# of positives exposed / all exposed

# of positives *not* exposed / all not exposed

**What is the mean and standard deviation for the Wechsler IQ test?**

**Mean = 100**
**Standard deviation = 15**

(This never changes – the test is re-normed periodically so that whatever the population's average IQ is always equals 100 on the test)

**How much of a population (assuming a "normal" distribution) is included in one standard deviation from the mean?**

**Approximately 68 %**

(34 % in each standard deviation, on each side of the average)

**How much of a population (assuming a normal distribution) is included in two standard deviations from the mean?**

**Almost everyone!**

**Approximately 95–96 %** (depending on rounding)

*(You will note that a 95 % confidence interval is approximately the same as quoting two standard deviations from the mean.)*

What is the "validity" of a test?

Whether the test succeeds in measuring what it is supposed to measure

What is the reliability of a test?

How similar the results of the test would be, if it could be repeated in the same population & way over & over

(Also used to mean whether similar results are obtained in multiple uses of a real world instrument in different settings.)

**What is a type 1 error?**

**The kind the experimenter "wants" to make – finding a difference when there wasn't anything there**

**What is a type 2 error?**

**Opposite of a type 1 – Failing to find a difference that was really there**

**What are the other names for type 1 and type 2 errors?**

**Alpha & beta errors (respectively)**

**How do you remember which is which, between alpha & beta errors?**

**All the dogs want to be the "alpha dog" – the one in charge**

**Alpha errors are the type we'd all like to make as researchers – in favor of our idea** (hypothesis)

How do I know if a study is retrospective?

If it looks at data that was collected *before* the study was designed, it's retrospective!

Example: Today, we decide to conduct a study using data from the 1980s, to see how many 15-year-olds were smoking, at that time.

| | |
|---|---|
| Why do we care if a study was retrospective, or not? | It is a weaker design – we should be a little less certain of the results |
| | It can be difficult to get accurate information from the past, and the data collection is prone to bias. |
| What is a longitudinal design? | One that follows the subjects forward in time, often for long periods of time |
| | *(such as the Framingham heart disease study, for example)* |
| What is a cross-sectional study design? | One that looks at just one point in time, usually comparing two or more groups |
| | Example: What percentage of 15-year-olds from various ethnic groups in the USA are smoking cigarettes during a 1-month data collection period. |
| What is a case–control study? | A study in which each research subject is matched to a control with the same characteristics |
| | (For example, research subjects with lung cancer are matched with a control who does not have lung cancer, but does have the same age, ethnicity, & occupation.) |
| What is a cohort study? | A study comparing two groups that have certain things of interest in common (aka cohorts) |
| | (For example, you study children taught with one reading method to children taught with a different method. You then follow school achievement, to see whether on method seems to produce better outcomes than the other.) |
| **What does the "p-value" tell you?** | **The probably that the result you're looking at is "real," and not due to chance** |

**What p-value is typically used to separate statistically significant results from statistically not significant results?**

**95 % or p < 0.05**

What's so magical about 95 % certainty, why not 92.68 %?

95 % was given as an example in the original statistical article, and completely unintentionally on the author's part, it stuck!

Is a p-value of <0.01 more significant than a p of <0.05?

Yes –
< 1 % probability that the result was due to chance, is better than 5 %, right?

**If you obtain a p-value of 0.021, you have a statistically significant result, because it is less than 0.05. How can you specifically interpret the p-value, though?**

**2.1 % of the time, the result you found in the study will occur by chance**

**Is statistical significance the same as clinical significance?**

**No –**
**Clinically significant results should also be statistically significant BUT many statistically significant results may not clinically important**

Why would a statistically significant result *not* be clinically significant?

Usually because the "effect size" is very small –
So clinically there isn't a big effect on the patient, even though the result is so consistent, or the sample size so large, that it is statistically significant

(Example: Suppose a study shows that changing the diet causes a 0.03 change in the INR very reliably. If the result is consistent &/or the sample size large, the result is likely to be significant. Such a small change, though, is not clinically of interest.)

**What is a meta-analysis?**

**Putting together a group of already completed studies and analyzing them together**

| | |
|---|---|
| **Why do people do meta-analyses?** | **Usually to get a much larger sample size than any of the studies can provide alone** |
| **Are meta-analyses a good way to strengthen results?** | **In some ways, yes –**<br>**But there are many difficulties with combining data "after the fact" that can make their results inconclusive** |
| How is a systematic review different from a meta-analysis? | The review tried to be comprehensive & to apply strict criteria to evaluating the methods used & results obtained by different studies – IT DOES NOT, though, combine the data of different studies to produce new results!!! |
| **Is it a good idea to have a wide variety of people included in a study?** | **That depends –**<br>**The study group should be as much like the group you want to use the results with as possible** |
| **What is it called when we apply results from a study to people out in the real population?** | **Generalizing –**<br>We're only supposed to "generalize" to populations that match the one in the study, officially<br><br>*Generalization to another population is NOT valid* |
| **If you are having trouble with a statistical calculation on the exam, what is a good strategy to make the numbers you should use clearer to you?** | **Make a 2 × 2 table (if the data match that pattern)**<br>• **Put "normal" & "abnormal result" on one axis (row or column)**<br>• **Put "disease" & "no disease" on the other (column or row)** |
| What is "attributable risk" (AR) and how do you calculate it? | – The difference between the risk of disease in a group of interest, compared to the risk in a comparison group<br><br>– simple subtraction<br><br>Example: risk of lung cancer in smokers – risk in nonsmokers = attributable risk (AR) |

| | |
|---|---|
| What is the "absolute risk reduction" statistic (ARR)? How is it calculated? | – The amount of risk *removed* by the treatment or intervention |
| | – simple subtraction |
| | Example: Risk of children dying after acquiring measles in a particular nation – the same risk if the children are supplemented with vitamin A = absolute risk reduction (ARR) |
| What does the "power calculation" tell you? | The likelihood of finding the result, if it is really present |
| How is the power calculation done? | Power = $1 - \beta$ (Beta is the probability of making a type II error – missing the result you were looking for, when it was really there.) |
| In general, how can you increase the power of a study? | Add subjects |
| | Look for a larger difference between the conditions (larger differences are easier to detect than small ones) |
| | Use a better, more consistent, measuring instrument |
| What is the "precision" of a test? | How reliably or consistently it measures something |
| | *(In other words, if your test could measure the same thing in the same conditions over & over, it should always get the same result, if it is very precise.)* |
| What is the "accuracy" of a test, then? | Generally used to mean how *valid* is the test – is it measuring what it was meant to measure? |
| How is NNT, number needed to treat, calculated & what does it tell you? | On the average, how many patients must you treat (with a particular intervention) for one patient to benefit? |
| | $1 \div ARR = NNT$ |
| | (ARR stands for absolute risk reduction) |

| | |
|---|---|
| How is the NNH, number needed to **harm**, calculated & what does it tell you? | On the average, how many people must be exposed to a risk for one person to be harmed?<br><br>$1 \div AR = NNH$<br><br>(AR is attributable risk) |
| What is selection bias in medical research? | When the way subjects are assigned to different study groups creates differences between the groups |
| What is lead-time bias? | Findings are biased due to earlier detection of a particular disease<br><br>(Generally it is a bias that shows improved survival with a new intervention. The effect is really due to earlier detection of the problem with the new intervention, not due to an improvement in the disease process or outcome) |
| What is the observer-expectancy effect? | The expectations of the researcher *cause* results to shift in the direction he or she expects (via various mechanisms) |
| What is the Hawthorne effect in research? | A finding that results *from the experience of being studied*, rather than from the item or intervention being studied |
| **What is "publication bias?"** | **The tendency for positive results to be published much more often than negative results** |
| What has been done to reduce publication bias? | Clinical trial registries –<br>Checking the registry tells you which studies were registered, but not what results their results, so it is only a partial solution |
| What is length bias, also known as survival bias? | Patient groups may be biased toward the healthier or longer living patients, because there are simply more of those patients available for enrollment<br><br>(survival & other variables being studied are then overestimated, because the sickest patients died too rapidly to be part of the study) |

| | |
|---|---|
| When does attrition bias affect study results? | Attrition bias occurs when the patients who drop out of the study, or those lost to follow-up, are different from those that stayed |
| There are two types of "recall bias." What are they & how can they affect results? | Recency effect – more recent events tend to be reported more or better |
| | Content effect – certain types of content may be remembered better or more easily, so that a false impression of *the overall* events that actually occurred |
| What is response bias? | The tendency for certain types of information to be reported, and other omitted |
| | (For example, a patient might avoid giving information about sensitive or stigmatizing experiences, such as STDs, but be very interested in reporting an important emotional event, such as a birth experience.) |
| In general, should you use t-tests to compare more than two different mean (average) values? | No – Each *t*-test you do has risks for error, so doing a lot of t-tests means lots of chance for error |
| If you need to compare a lot of different means, is there a test that lets you look at all of the differences, but just doing the test one time, so your chances of error happen just one time? | Yes! – An example is the ANOVA. Multiple means can be compared by running just this one test |
| The "odds ratio" statistic is most classically used with which design? | Case–control studies (comparing one "case" to a matched control) |
| The "relative risk" statistic is similar. It is most classically associated with which study design? | Cohort studies (comparing multiple groups or "cohorts" of people) |
| The case–control design is useful in epidemiology to search for what information? | Exposure issue or risk factor for development of disease |

Generally, a case–control design compares which two groups of people?

Those with the disease or characteristic are compared to a group without it

The prevalence of a disease can be rapidly collected using what sort of design?

Cross-sectional

(Prevalence is existing cases of a disease present in the population)

To find the incidence of a disease, what general sort of disease would you usually need to use?

Prospective

(how many new cases appear in the population, over a defined time period)

Although a cross-sectional study could tell you the prevalence of a disease, and risk factors associated with the disease, what question is it *unable* to answer?

Causality –

You can see what is there, but you cannot be certain why it's there or how it got there

If you would like to know which therapy is best for a particular disorder, what is the rank order for preferred study designs?

Generally it is:
Randomized controlled trial
Cohort
Case control

Generally speaking, what is the best design to see whether a new diagnostic tool is useful?

Prospective & blinded comparison to a gold standard

Generally speaking, what is the best design to learn whether a new physical exam technique should be adopted?

Prospective & blinded comparison to the gold standard

Randomized controlled trials are generally considered the best technique for what sorts of questions in medicine?

Best therapy
Best prevention
Etiology or harm of treatment

(Meta-analysis & Systematic review are also useful for these topics)

| | |
|---|---|
| In general, the hierarchy of research designs, as used in medicine, puts the designs in what order (from most powerful to least)? | Randomized control trial (RCT)<br><br>Cohort<br><br>Case–control<br><br>Case series<br><br>(Meta-analysis & systematic reviews can sometimes substitute for randomized control trials, although they are not fully equal.) |
| In the case of a study about prognosis, RCTs are usually not possible. Which designs are preferred (and in what rank order)? | Cohort<br><br>Case–control<br><br>Case series |
| Why is blinding important, and what does "triple" blinding mean? | Blinding reduces possibilities for bias<br>Triple blinding is:<br><br>**Researcher** does not know intervention (removes observer-expectancy bias)<br><br>**Patient** doesn't know intervention (removes bias due to their expectations)<br><br>**Data recorder/analyzer** doesn't know hypothesis (removed bias due to their wishes or expectations) |
| Why are the results from cohort studies considered less reliable from those of randomized control trials (RCTs)? | It is possible that the cohorts differ in important ways *other than the variable under study*<br><br>This creates a possible "confounder" – meaning that findings may be due to unmeasured differences between the groups, rather than the reflecting the variable under study |
| What is a "confounder?" | A confounder is an unmeasured variable that differs between the group being studied & the group being compared *that actually accounts for the findings!*<br><br>So it appears the findings are due to the variable being studied, when they are actually due to the (unmeasured & unknown) confounder |

Although there are other options, the main ways to control for confounding in medical research are _____, _____ & _____?

Randomization
*(in assignment of patients or subjects to conditions)*

Elimination of bias

&

Adequate sample size
*(determined by your power calculation)*

Why are the findings from a case–control study considered less reliable than the findings from a cohort study (or RCT)?

Because statistically significant findings are associations only. Causality cannot be determined.

Do case series have any value?

Yes, especially in rare disorders with a very small potential patient population.

We can still gain knowledge from them, but it is difficult to interpret, because there is no comparison or control group.

What is an "intention to treat" analysis?

An analysis that includes all available patient data according to the group the patient was randomized to – regardless of whether the patient actually stopped treatment, crossed over to treatment, was lost to follow-up, etc.

What is the importance of using an "intention-to-treat" (ITT) analysis?

It is a conservative measure of how successful a treatment under study is, because some of the patients in both the control & experimental groups are actually members of the opposite group (in terms of what treatment they received, in reality).

In other words, if you do an RCT with ITT, and you still get an effect, you can be fairly certain that you've found an important difference!

What problems in research designs is ITT analysis meant to address?

Noncompliance by subjects

&

Lost to follow-up subjects

# Chapter 7
# General Rheumatology Question and Answer Items

What is the new name for juvenile rheumatoid arthritis?

Juvenile idiopathic arthritis (JIA)

What is required to make a diagnosis of JIA, in terms of age & duration of symptoms?

Began before 16 years old

Arthritis in at least one joint lasting more than 6 weeks

What are the three types of JIA?

1. Oligoarticular (few joints – <4)
2. Polyarticular (many joints – >4)
3. Systemic (spikes fevers)

(Remember this is based on the presentation in the first 6 months for the polyarticular form)

What is the old name for oligoarticular JIA?

"pauci" articular JIA

(same meaning, terminology just adjusted)

**How is polyarticular juvenile idiopathic arthritis (JIA) determined?**

**Presentation in the first 6 months after onset of the disorder**

**Systemic arthritis is most likely an autoimmune disorder. Which cytokines are especially important in "systemic" JIA?**

IL-6 & IL-1

© Springer Science+Business Media New York 2015
C.M. Houser, *Pediatric Tricky Topics, Volume 1*,
DOI 10.1007/978-1-4939-1859-1_7

**What is the characteristic pain/
activity pattern for JIA?
    (2 aspects)**

**Morning stiffness that improves with
daytime activity**

&

*Worsens* **following rest!**

**Is loss of developmental
milestones a feature of JIA?**

**It can be**

(if pain or joint changes without pain limit
the child's physical capabilities)

In oligoarthritis JIA, do most
children present with large joint
involvement, or is it small joints?

Large joints

**Positive ANA is most common
in which sort of JIA?**

**Oligoarticular**

How can you remember that ANA
mainly goes with oligoarticular
JIA?

Think of a girl named ANA, who has her
name printed on her T-shirt, sitting on a chair
with a swollen knee and elbow

**Are oligoarticular JIA patients
likely to have a positive
rheumatoid factor?**

**No.**

**(Aside from elevated ANA, the other
studies are usually normal)**

**Which patients with pediatric
arthritis are at highest risk for
uveitis & the related
complications?**

**Oligoarticular JIA & psoriatic arthritis**

Why are the ophthalmological
complications of oligoarticular
JIA a big deal?

Uveitis can lead to cataracts, glaucoma, &
blindness

(many uveitis patients are asymptomatic,
but need to be closely monitored for ocular
damage)

If a patient with polyarticular JIA
has facial growth abnormalities,
how might that be related
to the JIA?

Polyarticular can affect the axial skeleton –
temporomandibular joint involvement can
lead to micrognathia

**Although positive rheumatoid factor only occurs in about 10 % of polyarticular JIA patients, what is its significance?**

**Bad prognosis – aggressive management will be needed**

**(likely to persist into adulthood)**

How can you remember that RF is associated with polyarticular JIA?

It's RuF (rough) to have so many joints affected

**Uveitis is a common complication of what type of JIA?**

**Oligoarticular**

**(especially in females with + *ANA*)**

**Which HLA type is associated with psoriatic arthritis & enthesitis-related arthritis (such as ankylosing spondylitis)?**

**HLA – B27**

**Arthritis with anemia, but elevated white count and platelets suggests what diagnosis?**

**JIA**

**Arthritis with leukopenia & a photosensitive rash suggests which rheumatological diagnosis?**

**Systemic lupus erythematosus (SLE)**

What are the typical ages of onset for the types of JIA?

Overall there are two peaks:
1–3 years & adolescence

(*polyarticular* has both peaks,
*systemic* is spread evenly across the age groups,
*oligoarticular* has just the early age peak 1–3 years)

(onset must be before age 16 to consider it any sort of JIA, though)

What is the typical age of onset for enthesitis-related arthritis is _____?

10–12 years

| | |
|---|---|
| Like oligoarticular JIA, psoriatic arthritis typically begins in which age group? | 1–3 years |
| **Which gender is most likely to develop JIA?** | **Females** |
| **What physical findings are expected in systemic JIA?** **(4)** | **Spiking fevers** **Lymphadenopathy/HSM** **Salmon-colored morbilliform rash** **Arthritis (of course)** |
| **What is the first-line treatment for JIA?** | **NSAIDs** (physical therapy is also helpful) |
| **What sorts of medications are second-line treatment for JIA?** | **Steroids & Immunosuppressants** |
| **If a child has systemic JIA, is the prognosis better when few joints, or many joints, are involved?** | **Few** |
| **Although it is unusual to have a positive rheumatoid factor with oligoarticular disease, what does it mean for prognosis when it's positive?** | **Bad prognosis** |
| RF+ JIA is most often seen in which age & gender group? | Adolescent females |
| **Aside from uveitis, is it a good or bad prognostic to have a positive ANA with oligoarticular JIA?** | **Good** |
| **It is unusual for JIA patients to have a positive rheumatoid factor. Which type of JIA is most likely to have a positive RF?** | **Polyarticular** **(Bad prognostic)** |

| | |
|---|---|
| Is a positive ANA a good or bad prognostic for any type of JIA patient? | **Good** (relatively common in both pauci and polyarticular disease, but most common in oligoarticular patients) |
| How common is systemic JIA? | **Fairly uncommon – About 10 % of JIA patients** |
| How many joints are affected in systemic JIA? | **Variable** |
| What types of joints are affected in systemic JIA? | **Any type can be affected** |
| Uveitis and mucosal ulcers (oral and urethral), make up the findings in what rheumatological syndrome? | **Behcet's** (arthralgia, but not generally arthritis, is also seen) |
| Is the constellation of uveitis with oral & genital ulcers associated with a particular HLA type? | **Yes.** **HLA – B51 (Behcet's syndrome)** |
| How can you remember the antibodies that go with Sjogren's syndrome? | **Sjogren's patients have irritated eyes – they might "RoLa" eyes in annoyance with all the burning & itching** |
| What is the main problem in Sjogren's syndrome? | **Everything is dry – glands are infiltrated with lymphocytes –Dry eyes, dry mouth** |
| How is Sjogren's syndrome treated? | **Immunosuppressants/corticosteroids and** *artificial tears* (good oral hygiene also helpful) |
| How is a Sjogren's syndrome diagnosis confirmed? | Lip or salivary gland biopsy |
| What two preliminary tests are often used when a diagnosis of Sjogren's is suspected? | **ESR (elevated) & Schirmer test (measures amount of tear production)** Mnemonic: "Schirmer" sounds like "swimmer." Reminds you that the "swimmer" test measures $H_2O$ in the eye! |

| | |
|---|---|
| Is the glandular infiltration by lymphocytes in Sjogren's syndrome painful? | No – the glands sometimes enlarge, but it is painless enlargement |
| In general terms, what causes Henoch-Schonlein purpura (HSP)? | **Autoimmune vasculitis (specifically, an IgA-related leukocytoclastic vasculitis)** *leukocytoclastic vasculitis means that neutrophils invade & do damage to the (small) vessels* |
| What are the usual triggers for HSP? | **Viral infections or Grp A strep** (other bacterial infections can also act as triggers) |
| What is the characteristic pattern for the rash of HSP? | **Dependent areas – usually buttocks and lower extremities** |
| HSP patients have purpura – do they have thrombocytopenia? | No |
| In addition to the skin rash, what other organ systems are often affected when HSP occurs? | **Renal GI Joints (& occasionally CNS)** |
| In addition to hematuria, what other renal problems do HSP patients sometimes develop? | **Glomerulonephritis & Nephrotic syndrome (in some cases, renal insufficiency or failure & renal-related hypertension)** |
| What are HSP's main GI symptoms & signs? | **Pain, vomiting, & bleeding** |
| HSP patients are at risk for what serious cause of episodic abdominal pain? | **Intussusception** (vasculitic lesions in the gut can serve as a lead point) |
| What is the prognosis for patients with HSP? | **Great – goes away in 4–6 weeks** |

| | |
|---|---|
| Does HSP require treatment? | No – supportive care & removal of suspected triggers, when possible |
| | Steroids & other immunosuppressants are sometimes used, especially for severe disease, but current evidence regarding efficacy is not adequate for a clear answer. |
| | *(short-term prednisone has not been shown to improve renal disease)* |
| **What muscle symptoms do patients with dermatomyositis complain of?** | **Weakness (mainly in the proximal muscles)** |
| Will dermatomyositis patients have elevated CK? | Yes (the problem is in the muscle, not in the nerves innervating them – this means CK will be up) |
| **Does dermatomyositis present acutely or gradually?** | **Gradual onset** |
| **What are the two "famous" buzzword findings associated with dermatomyositis?** | **1. Heliotrope rash (purplish rash around the eyes)**<br>**2. Gottron papules over the small joints of the hands (looks like a red rash)** |
| **What nail finding goes with dermatomyositis?**<br>  **(2)** | **Nailbed telangiectasias**<br><br>    &<br><br>**Periungual erythema** |
| **How do infants develop neonatal systemic lupus erythematosus?** | **Antibodies passed from Mom to fetus – especially in mothers carrying anti-Ro/SSA antibodies**<br><br>**(Not all of the Moms who pass the antibodies are known to have lupus, however. Some develop it later, but not all of them.)** |
| **Do infants with neonatal SLE have any characteristic skin findings?** | **Yes –**<br>**Scaly, red, annular rash *on face & upper body*** |
| | 70 % will have skin findings – 2/3 of those will have skin findings at birth, the rest develop over the first few months of life |

| | |
|---|---|
| Aside from skin changes, should you expect other findings on physical exam of an infant with neonatal SLE? | Hepatosplenomegaly |
| **What is the natural course of neonatal SLE?** | **Resolves over time (except for the most serious problem)** |
| **What consequence of neonatal SLE can be life threatening to the infant?** | **Heart block**<br><br>**This problem will not resolve, and often requires cardiac pacing** |
| **What are the possible cardiac effects of neonatal SLE? (3)** | **Pericarditis/myocarditis**<br><br>**Cardiomyopathy & heart failure**<br><br>**Heart block** |
| How common is it for infants with neonatal SLE to have cardiac effects? | Common – about 2/3 will have them |
| Children and adults with SLE often have hematological changes. Are any hematological changes seen in neonatal SLE? | Yes – near pancytopenia with anemia, thrombocytopenia, and neutropenia |
| **How is neonatal SLE treated?** | **Steroids, if needed**<br>**Pacing, if needed**<br>**Otherwise supportive** |
| What is the other name for the anti-Ro and anti-La antibodies, respectively? | Anti-SSA<br>Anti-SSB |
| SLE is more common in African Americans than it is in Caucasians. Is there an increased incidence in any other ethnic groups? | Yes – nearly all of them (Native American, Asian, & Hispanic) |
| **In which body cavities do lupus patients tend to build up fluid where it doesn't belong?** | **Pericardial sac & pleural membranes** |

| | |
|---|---|
| **In addition to the butterfly malar rash, what other skin abnormalities are common with lupus?** (2) | **Photosensitivity** & **Discoid lesions** |
| If lupus affects the CNS, what sorts of problems does it create? | Many, the most common are – Headaches (including migraine) Neuropsych syndromes Seizures |
| How many neuropsychiatric syndromes are associated with SLE, in the current SLE case definitions? *Note: This is a change!* | Nineteen – Previously only seizures & psychosis were included |
| What sorts of problems is the peripheral nervous system vulnerable to, with SLE? | Demyelinating disorders Peripheral neuropathies |
| **What are the main complications of SLE?** (5) | 1. **Renal failure** 2. **Increased infections** 3. **Cardiovascular disease** 4. **Neurological problems** 5. **Clot-related problems** |
| **Why might SLE patients have lowered immunity to infections?** | **Leukopenia & lymphopenia** + **immunosuppressant medications** |
| **How is SLE treated?** | **Steroids, Hydroxychloroquine, & Cyclophosphamide (for severe disease)** |
| What are spondyloarthropathies? | Ankylosing spondylitis Reactive arthritis (previously Reiter's syndrome) Enteropathic arthritis (IBD related) Psoriatic arthritis |

| | |
|---|---|
| **How can you differentiate general low back pain due to muscle strain from the low back pain of the spondyloarthropathies?** | **Spondyloarthropathies get *better with movement & worse with rest*** |
| **What other body system is sometimes affected in spondyloarthropathy patients?** | **The eye (uveitis/iritis)**<br><br>**(Uveitis/iritis is seen with most HLA-B27 related disorders)** |
| Are the ulcers of Behcet's syndrome painful? | Yes (both in the mouth and on the genitals) |
| Is belly pain a part of Behcet's syndrome? | It can be – GI ulcerations also occur |
| Other than the funny appearance, will kids with dermatomyositis complain about the rash? | Often, yes – it can be itchy |
| **What sort of symptoms does the proximal muscle weakness of dermatomyositis cause?**<br>    **(3 categories)** | **"Clumsiness"**<br><br>**Difficulty climbing stairs or rising from chairs**<br>**Difficulty dressing**<br><br>**Difficulty swallowing or voice change** |
| **What cutaneous-related finding causes significant morbidity in dermatomyositis?** | **Calcinosis cutis –**<br>**Calcium deposits in the skin linked to pain, skin ulceration & atrophy, nerve entrapment & contractures**<br><br>**(1/3 of patients develop calcinosis cutis)** |
| **How do dermatomyositis patients present, overall?** | **Rash**<br>**Proximal muscle weakness**<br>**Myalgia & athralgias** |
| **How is dermatomyositis treated?** | **High-dose steroids**<br>**Immunosuppressants including methotrexate & cyclophosphamide**<br>**IVIG** |

| | |
|---|---|
| What environmental exposure is a problem for dermatomyositis patients? | Sunlight (photosensitive)<br><br>*Must use sunscreen to avoid burns, worsening rash, & sometimes also worsening muscle weakness!* |
| **Reactive arthritis (previously called Reiter syndrome) is highly associated with chlamydial infections in adolescents & adults. In kids, which infectious agents are more common triggers?** | **Enteric pathogens (Yersinia, Shigella, Salmonella, & Campylobacter typically)**<br><br>(FYI – Giardia, & C. diff can also trigger it) |
| **What is the famous mnemonic for reactive arthritis?** | **"Can't see,<br>   can't pee,<br>     can't climb a tree."** |
| How long after the trigger infection does reactive arthritis usually appear? | 1–4 weeks |
| Which of the pediatric rheumatological diseases are more common in males? | Enthesitis-related arthritis &<br>Reactive arthritis<br>Behcet's syndrome (depending on location)<br><br>(the others are generally more common in females) |
| **Why might a juvenile systemic sclerosis (commonly known as scleroderma) patient have pulmonary complaints?** | **It can invade the lungs, causing pulmonary fibrosis** |
| What are the most common types of systemic sclerosis in children? | Diffuse cutaneous systemic sclerosis<br><br>&<br><br>Localized scleroderma (aka morphea) |
| **What is the most typical presentation for a scleroderma patient?** | **Raynaud's syndrome (fingers that turn white, then blue, then red)**<br><br>*Not all Raynaud's patients have scleroderma, however!* |

If an ichthyosis patient is diagnosed at birth, and later is found to have intellectual disability with spastic limbs, what syndrome might that be?

Sjogren-Larsson Syndrome

(autosomal recessive disorder of lipid metabolism – not related to regular Sjogren's at all)

**What is "serositis?"**

**Pericarditis, peritonitis, and/or pleuritis (seen with SLE – any one or more of the three may be seen)**

**If SLE is suspected, but you check the ANA and it is negative, what should you conclude?**

**Probably not lupus.**

What systemic complaints do SLE patients often have?

Fatigue, malaise, weight loss, fever

**What is the most *sensitive* test for SLE?**

**ANA – it is good for screening because it is sensitive, but there will be many false positives**

**What is the most *specific* test for lupus?**

**Anti-Smith antibody**

**In addition to scleroderma, which other rheumatological disorder very often has Raynaud's phenomenon as part of the disorder?**

**SLE**

**Which antibodies cause heart block in neonatal SLE?**

**Anti-Ro (also known as anti-SSA)**

**Why would a lupus patient have a seizure?**

**Lupus cerebritis – Vasculitis affecting the brain**

**If a patient has rheumatological complaints or findings, and an *autoimmune hemolytic anemia*, which rheumatological disorder should you think of?**

**SLE**

(can also have anemia of chronic disease)

| | |
|---|---|
| **What is the second-line treatment for mild SLE, if NSAIDs are not sufficient?** | **Hydroxychloroquine (Plaquenil™)** |
| What are the main side effects of the second-line treatment for SLE? | Ocular complaints (blurring & retinal damage) & ototoxicity |
| **What commonly occurs when tapering SLE steroid doses?** | **Flare-up of the disease symptoms**<br><br>**(usually not a reason to increase the steroids, though)** |
| How long after infection with Lyme disease will serum antibody be detectable? What does this mean for testing? | 4–6 weeks<br><br>Expect negative results early in the disease & treat clinically |
| If a patient is being treated for Lyme disease, and suddenly develops fever, shaking chills, and back pain, what should you suspect? | Jarisch-Herxheimer reaction – supportive care will get the patient through it<br><br>(caused by lysis of the little critters with successful treatment – historically seen with syphilis treatment) |
| **It is common for the boards to present cases with a positive rheumatoid factor. Should you rely on that as an indicator of JIA?** | **No – not reliable** |
| **If the boards describes a child with a limp due to leg pain that is "worse at night," and without any joint swelling or rash, what are they probably describing?** | **Growing pains** |
| **A child is described with frequent joint sprains and "loose joints." What should you suspect?** | **Hypermobility – counsel regarding stretching and appropriate sport activities, but no treatment needed** |
| **When are steroids typically used in the treatment of JIA?** | **Cardiac involvement or failure with NSAID regimens** |

**When are steroids typically used in the treatment of JIA?**

**For quick improvement if NSAID regimens have failed**

**What is the usual NSAID regimen for JIA treatment?**

**M Melixicam**
**I Ibuprofen**
**N Naproxen**

How is the pain of acute leukemia different from the pain of JIA?

Acute leukemia wakes the patient at night, and is not focused on a joint

**What is the eponymic name for systemic JIA?**

**Still's disease**

(can also occur in adults, but then it's "adult-onset Still's disease)

What is the typical age for a Kawasaki's patient?

18–24 months

Do Kawasaki's patients have a positive ANA?

No

**What GU symptom sometimes occurs with Kawasaki's?**

**Sterile pyuria**

(white cells in the urine without bacteria)

How can Kawasaki's affect the CNS?

Seizures and meningitis (aseptic)

**What is the typical CBC for a Kawasaki's patient?**

**High white count**
**High platelets (especially ≥7 days after onset)**

**Aspirin is one part of the treatment of Kawasaki's. How long should a child with Kawasaki's continue ASA?**

**1–2 months –**

**Initially high dose (80 mg/kg/day) then low dose (5 mg/kg/day)**

Which joints typically swell in Henoch-Schonlein Purpura (HSP)?

Knees and ankles

**What is the nature of the joint involvement in HSP?**

**It is "periarticular," meaning that it affects the tissue around the joints primarily, rather than the joint itself**

**What is the buzzword for the skin lesions of HSP?**

**Palpable purpura**

**(think of the vasculitis inflaming & fluffing up the vessels – that's why you can feel it)**

**Which rheumatological condition tends to cause *ileoileal* intussusception?**

**HSP**

**(often harder to diagnose & correct, due to location)**

How common is renal involvement in HSP?

About 50 %
(but not necessarily very bad renal involvement)

**Granulomatosis with polyangiitis (formerly known as Wegener's granulomatosis) is most common in which ethnic group?**

**Caucasians**

A 9-year-old boy presents with rash, fever, and arthralgias a few weeks after he was successfully treated for a snake bite. What is wrong with him?

Serum sickness

(Type 3 hypersensitivity reaction – antivenins sometimes induce this response)

What is the most common organism to cause septic arthritis in kids older than 2 years?

Staph aureus

**If the boards presents a single, inflamed joint, and you can't tell whether it's septic arthritis or not, what should you do?**

**When in doubt, or if it can't be determined from the info given, treat for septic arthritis**
**(there is no time to lose – the board wants to make sure that you know this)**

**If you suspect rheumatic fever on the boards, what *must be* confirmed?**

**Documented history of strep infection**

If a child has a negative rapid strep test, does this rule-out a recent strep infection/rheumatic fever?

No

**What are acceptable ways to document strep infection?**

ASO titer or streptozyme (& culture, of course)

Emotional lability, along with purposeless rapid movements and muscle weakness, following an upper respiratory infection, suggests what diagnosis?

Sydenham's chorea (complication of strep infection)

**How is the arthritis of rheumatic fever most likely to be described?**

"Migratory"

**The most common murmur associated with rheumatic fever is "heard best at the apex." What is the lesion?**

Mitral valve regurgitation

**If a rheumatic fever patient develops a new murmur and mild CHF, what is the likely lesion?**

Aortic regurg/insufficiency

**Along with a documented Group A strep infection, what else is required to make a diagnosis of rheumatic fever?**

Jones criteria –

2 major or
1 major & 2 minor

Is arthritis a major or a minor criterion in the Jones system?

Major

**What about arthralgia? How does that fit in the Jones criteria?**

It is a *minor* criterion

**What are the minor criteria in the Jones system for rheumatic fever?**
**(5)**

The usual vague-type signs (except for the cardiac one):

1. **Fever**
2. **Arthralgia**
3. **Elevated acute phase reactants (ESR, CRP, etc.)**
4. **Prior rheumatic fever or heart disease**
5. **Prolonged PR interval** (*this one's unusual!*)

| | |
|---|---|
| **What are the major criteria in the Jones system?** | **CH = chorea**<br>**A = arthritis**<br>**N = nodules (subQ)**<br>**C = carditis**<br>**E = erythema marginatum (rash)** |
| How long does a rheumatic fever episode last? | 1 week to 1 month |
| In this era of antibiotic overuse, how can patients still end up with rheumatic fever? | 1. Foreign born<br>2. Sometimes the initial throat infection isn't noticed |
| **How is rheumatic fever treated?** | **Aspirin**<br><br>**(antibiotics are also routinely given, to decrease transmission)** |
| **If rheumatic fever is affecting the heart, what is the most appropriate treatment?** | **Steroids**<br>**(especially in cases of heart failure!)** |
| How is Sydenham's chorea treated?<br>    (2 ways) | Rest in a quiet (not stimulating) environment<br>Valproic acid for sedation (if needed) |
| **What is the long-term outcome for joints in rheumatic fever?** | **The arthritis resolves between episodes** |
| If arthritis is due to trauma, and you tap the joint, what will the fluid look like? | Clear or bloody (few WBCs) |
| **Which type of arthritis has a low glucose in the joint fluid?** | **Bacterial (aka septic)** |
| **What is the normal appearance of synovial fluid?** | **Clear to straw-colored (but easy to see through)** |
| **Can synovial fluid have a white count of 20,000 and still be inflammatory rather than septic?** | **Yes, definitely.** |

| | |
|---|---|
| A 6-year-old female presents with joint pain and swelling, proteinuria, hematuria, crampy belly pain, and heme positive stools. She recently had a URI. What is the likely diagnosis? | Henoch-Schonlein purpura |
| A 7-year-old boy presents with joint pain after a recent URI. He has a new heart murmur, and he says the joints that hurt keep "moving around," What is his diagnosis? | Rheumatic fever (Documented Group A Strep infection needed, though) |
| **A migratory, macular rash develops on a child with a fever. It has discrete borders and is "salmon colored." It is on or near the torso. What rheumatology rash is it?** | **JIA** |
| Koebner phenomenon occurs in psoriasis. What does it mean when applied to the rash of JIA? | Minimal irritation of the skin results in appearance of the rash (same idea for both disorders) |
| Which is more common – oligoarticular or polyarticular JIA? | Oligoarticular – estimates from 30 to 60 % of patients<br><br>(Polyarticular = about 25 %, with 5 % RF positive & 20 % RF negative) |
| **What medication works well specifically for polyarticular JIA?** | **Anti-TNF treatments such as Etanercept (Enbrel®)** |
| **What two findings indicate a *worse overall prognostics* for JIA?** | **1. More severe at onset**<br>**2. Rheumatoid factor positive** |
| **What is macrophage activation syndrome?** | **A serious complication of JIA (& sometimes other rheumatic diseases) –**<br><br>**Elevated LFTs, pancytopenia, and bad coagulopathy, & neurological problems**<br><br>(a little bit like HELLP syndrome in pregnant patients) |

| | |
|---|---|
| How is macrophage activation syndrome treated? | Steroids and immunosuppressants <br><br> (Cyclosporin A is used in particular, don't use methotrexate) |
| **Inflammation of areas where tendons, ligaments, or fascia connect to bone has what special name?** | **Enthesitis** |
| Which rheumatologic disorders can be properly considered "enthesitis related arthritides?" | Juvenile ankylosing spondylitis <br> Juvenile psoriatic arthritis <br> IBD-related arthritis <br> Post-infectious reactive arthritides |
| IBD-related arthritides often respond well to which specific medication? | Infliximab (an anti-TNF agent) |
| **There are two patterns of arthritis associated with inflammatory bowel disease. What are they?** | **Peripheral & Axial** |
| **Which type of IBD-related arthritis is associated with HLA-B27?** | **The axial type** |
| **Which type of IBD-related arthritis occurs in conjunction with flares of the gut illness?** | **Peripheral <br> (Specifically, peripheral type 1, also known as oligoarticular)** |
| **Does psoriasis need to be present to diagnose psoriatic arthritis?** | **Oddly enough, no** |
| Where does psoriatic arthritis usually begin? | Finger joints <br> (dactylitis) |
| What are the two criteria for making a psoriatic arthritis diagnosis? | 1. Both psoriasis & arthritis are present <u>or</u> <br> 2. Arthritis is present + 2 of these: <br><br> Nail findings (pits) <br> Dactylitis (sausage digits) <br> 1st-degree relative with psoriasis |

**What is the relationship between the onset of arthritis and the onset of skin lesions on psoriasis?**

**Arthritis sometimes starts years before the skin findings**

The relationship between reactive arthritis and chlamydial infections is well-known. What gut infection is also a common trigger for reactive arthritis?

Campylobacter (both jejuni & coli)

**If a patient develops reactive arthritis after a GI infection, will he/she still have urethritis?**

**Yes.**

**What is the most commonly diagnosed vasculitis of childhood?**

**Henoch-Schonlein purpura**

**What is the second most commonly diagnosed vasculitis of childhood?**

**Kawasaki's**

**What is the mechanism of HSP?**    **IgA deposition in vessel walls**

**If a child develops HSP, you will need to check the urine, and a BUN & creatinine, to assess renal function. How long are children with HSP at risk for renal involvement?**

**At least 3 months after diagnosis(!)**

**The natural course of HSP is spontaneous resolution. What is the "trick" in making that statement?**

**40 % of patients have recurrences (up to 2 years after the initial episode)**

**What is the main cause of acquired heart disease in children (in the developed nations)?**

**Kawasaki's**

**What gall bladder complication sometimes develops with Kawasaki's disease?**

**Hydrops of the gall bladder (fluid in and about the gall bladder)**

| | |
|---|---|
| **Does rapid & appropriate treatment for Kawasaki's eliminate the risk of coronary aneurysms?** | **No –**<br>**About 4 % still develop aneurysms** |

| | |
|---|---|
| **Which Kawasaki's patients are at increased risk for development of coronary aneurysms?**<br>(5 factors, including:<br>**Demographics**<br>**Fever related**<br>**Pattern of disease or Treatment related**) | 1. **Males**<br>2. **<1 year old**<br>3. **Fever despite treatment**<br>4. **Recurrent Kawasaki's**<br>5. **Delay in treatment**<br><br>(there is some suggestion that older children, 9–17 years old, may also be at increased risk, along with certain ethnic groups, but the data is not yet clear) |

| | |
|---|---|
| **If you're giving IVIG, what side effects do you need to watch for?** | **Aseptic meningitis &**<br>**Anaphylaxis**<br>**(mainly seen in IgA deficient patients)**<br><br>*Also fluid overload in infants* |

| | |
|---|---|
| **What is the leading cause of death in Kawasaki's patients?** | **Myocardial infarction**<br>**(due to coronary aneurysms)** |

| | |
|---|---|
| **If a Kawasaki's patient is going to have serious cardiac complications, when do they typically occur?** | **In the first year following the illness** |

| | |
|---|---|
| **What is polyarteritis nodosa?** | **A vasculitis causing renal, skin, and musculoskeletal problems** |

| | |
|---|---|
| **What is the pathological process in polyarteritis nodosa?** | **Focal segmental necrotizing vasculitis – it goes after medium-sized vessels** |

| | |
|---|---|
| **What is the main, overall, complication polyarteritis causes?** | **Aneurysms**<br>**(of medium-sized vessels)** |

| | |
|---|---|
| **What very unusual, and important, finding can develop in polyarteritis nodosa patients *if there is a concurrent HepB infection?*** | **ORCHITIS!**<br><br>**(Imagine parts of the damaged liver falling off into the scrotum, the pressure causes necrosis of some of the testicular vessels, leading to orchitis!)** |

**What is the buzzword for the pathology you see with granulomatosis with polyangiitis (GPA), formerly known as Wegener's granulomatosis?**

**Necrotizing granulomatous vasculitis (At least it has "granulomatosis" in the name, right?)**

**Which organs does GPA affect?**

**Respiratory tree**
    **&**
**Kidneys**

**What kind of vessels does GPA damage?**

**Small vessels – and mainly in the respiratory tree or kidney**

How are vasculitides like "the three bears?"

Each one likes a particular sized vessel – much like the three bears each needed a different sized bowl of porridge

Large – Takayasu's – Papa Bear
Medium – Polyarteritis & Kawasaki's – Mama Bear
Small – Wegener's – Baby Bear

**Which marker is especially helpful in diagnosing GPA?**

**cANCA**

**What facial abnormality is a tipoff to GPA?**

**Saddle nose deformity –**
**Inflammation in the small vessels of the nose can damage the septum, leading to necrosis and saddle nose**

Symptoms from which organ system usually lead to a childhood diagnosis of GPA?

Respiratory tree
(usually precedes renal by several years – Epistaxis & hemoptysis especially common)

**How common is Takayasu's arteritis in the US population?**

**Rare**

**How common is Takayasu's in the pediatric population of Japan (or those of Japanese descent)?**

**Third most common vasculitis (after HSP & Kawasaki)**

Which ethnic groups are most likely to develop Behcet's disease?

Mediterranean or Far East heritage

| | |
|---|---|
| **In addition to oral and genital ulceration, what other skin lesions are common for Behcet patients?** | **Erythema nodosum**<br>**Necrotic folliculitis** |
| **Behcet disease patients often have a "positive pathergy test." What is that?** | **Prick skin with a needle –**<br>**Positive means that 48 h later the area will turn red, and form a papule or pustule** |
| Arthralgias are common in Behcet's syndrome. Is arthritis also common? | No – just arthralgias<br>(and sometimes rashes) |
| What is Behcet's syndrome? | A vasculitis |
| What is Takayasu's arteritis? | A vasculitis affecting large vessels (especially the aorta) |
| What proportion of SLE cases are diagnosed in people younger than 18 years old? | 1 in 5 |
| How likely is a pregnant woman to pass on neonatal SLE, if she is known to be positive for lupus by serology? | <10 % of infants will be affected |
| How common is it for SLE patients to have antiphospholipid antibodies? | About ½ have them |
| **Which antibodies are considered to be "antiphospholipid antibodies?"** | **Anticardiolipin**<br>**Lupus anticoagulant**<br>**B-2-glycoprotein-1** |
| **What complications are mainly associated with antiphospholipid antibodies?** | **Blood clots**<br>**Miscarriage**<br>**Thrombocytopenia** |
| What is the most common cause of the movement disorder "chorea," in children worldwide? | Post-streptococcal<br>(Sydenham's chorea) |
| **What hair problem is common with SLE?** | **Alopecia** |

In addition to SLE, what other rheumatologic disorder also causes a malar rash?

**Dermatomyositis**
**(although they usually also have the purplish heliotrope rash around the eyes to help you differentiate the two)**

In addition to arthritis, what other joint complication are lupus patients at increased to develop?

**Avascular necrosis – usually of the femoral head**

**(multiple causes – SLE itself, antiphospholipid antibodies, and steroid use)**

The joint disease of JIA and SLE look very similar, and both improve as the day goes by. Other than history, what will help you tell them apart?

SLE *does not* cause a destructive arthritis with joint changes on X-ray – JIA does

Antiphospholipid antibodies are associated with a lot of bad stuff. In addition to clots, chorea, & miscarriage, what other serious cardiovascular disorder are they related to?

**Libman-Sacks endocarditis**

The general class of medications used to treat lupus is _____?

**Antimalarials**
**(e.g., hydroxychloroquine)**

What are the main side-effects of steroids on the skeletal system?

**Avascular necrosis &**
**Osteopenia**
**(sometimes with fractures of long bones, or vertebral compression fractures)**

What are the main side effects of steroids on the endocrine system?

**Growth failure**
**Diabetes mellitus**
**(of course there are others – these are the main ones)**

What are the main side effects of steroids on the eyes?

**Glaucoma & cataracts**

What are the main side effects of steroids on the cardiovascular system?

**Hypertension & early atherosclerotic disease**

| | |
|---|---|
| What is "mixed connective tissue disease?" | A mix of dermatomyositis, lupus, and scleroderma |
| What patient population is most likely to develop mixed connective tissue disease? | Girls |
| **How do most cases of Sjogren's syndrome present in children?** | **Recurrent parotitis (painless) & keratoconjunctivitis sicca (dry, irritated eyes)** |
| **Although it is very uncommon, the boards would like you to know that Sjogren's patients are at increased risk for what malignancy?** | **Lymphoma (usually MALT lymphoma or non-Hodgkin's B-cell lymphomas)** |
| **What is _required_ to make a diagnosis of dermatomyositis?** | **Gottron papules or heliotrope rash (+4 associated lesser findings)**<br>• Lesser findings include proximal weakness, ↑ CPK, EMG or muscle biopsy findings, nondestructive arthritis, and anti-Jo-1 antibodies |
| Which diagnostic modality is in use for dermatomyositis diagnosis? | MRI (looking at changes in muscle tissue – increased T2) |
| **What is the main way to treat dermatomyositis?** | **High-dose steroids – typically prednisone 2 mg/kg/day**<br><br>**(Sun avoidance & methotrexate & immunosuppressants for muscle symptoms are also important)** |
| **What fingertip problem do children with scleroderma often develop?** | **Ulcerations (due to vascular insufficiency)** |
| **What is the usual sequence for Raynaud's syndrome?** | **Fingertips turn:**<br>**White (arterial spasm – no blood)**<br>**Blue (they've run out of oxygen)**<br>**Red (they're reperfusing)** |

**What is the other name for anti-topoisomerase antibodies, associated with scleroderma?**

**Anti-SCL-70 antibodies**

**Which internal organ system is most commonly affected by scleroderma?**

**GI**
**(especially distal esophagus/lower esophageal sphincter)**

**Can scleroderma affect the kidney?**

**It can – but usually as a consequence of hypertension**
(good HTN control has decreased the incidence of renal problems)

How is the prognosis for scleroderma patients with diffuse disease?

Poor

**What is the role of corticosteroids in scleroderma?**

*High dose is contraindicated!* – **can lead to renal crisis**

**If a scleroderma patient develops hypertension, which medication class has been found to be most helpful in avoiding long-term renal damage?**

**ACE inhibitors**

**What is the most common pediatric form of scleroderma, and what is its more common name?**

**Localized linear scleroderma – more commonly known as "morphea"**
(older name for it)

**What is the special term for linear scleroderma when it occurs on the face?**

*En coupe de sabre*
**"cut of the sword" – the lesion looks like the patient got a cut in a duel**

Is morphea/linear scleroderma limited to the skin?

Not always – it can extend to deeper tissues, or be primarily deep

(overlying skin may have a peau d'orange appearance)

Will linear scleroderma patients have serological markers of scleroderma?

No

**When does the pain of "growing pains" usually occur?**

**Evening or nighttime**

**What is a tipoff that leg pain is *not* due to growing pains, in terms of the timing and location of the pain?**

**Morning pain**
**Pain is in the joint**
**Pain is unilateral**

**Can growing pains limit a child's mobility?**

**No – if it does, it's something else**

Can growing pains wake children from sleep?

Yes
(but pain that wakes a child from sleep is still concerning)

By what age should growing pains disappear?

Thirteen

**If a child with hypermobility syndrome is symptomatic, what three interventions can you recommend for her?**
(Most patients are girls)

**NSAIDs**

**Physical therapy for muscle strengthening**

**Overall fitness improvement**

How do you test elbows & knees for hypermobility?

Extension beyond 10°
(test each side separately)

How do you test the thumb for hypermobility?

See if the patient can bend is the whole way back to the arm – like those kids at camp used to do!

How do you test the trunk for hyperextensibility?

Being able to flex to touch the floor with both palms, when the knees are straight

(better hope your patients aren't doing yoga, or they'll all qualify on this one)

If your patient can extend the hand and fingers, so that the fingers bend backwards to be parallel with the forearm, is this suspicious for hypermobility?

You bet it is

Why do we care whether patients have hypermobility syndrome?

1. Sometimes, they have joint pain
2. Sometimes, they have serious connective tissue disorders
(Ehlers-Danlos or Marfan's)

**How is Familial Mediterranean Fever treated?**

**Colchicine**

What are the symptoms of FMF, familial Mediterranean fever?

Recurring fevers lasting 5 h to 5 days, with abdominal pain
(may also have rash, arthritis, pleuritis, pericarditis, scrotal swelling)

Which ethnic group is most affected by Familial Mediterranean Fever?

East Mediterraneans –
Turkish, Armenian, certain Jewish populations

**What gene has been identified as the cause of familial Mediterranean fever?**

**"Pyrin" gene on chromosome 16**

**(it makes a protein that regulates certain inflammatory responses)**

**An 8-year-old child has a fever lasting longer than 5 days, pharyngitis, cervical adenitis, and aphthous stomatitis. There is no rash or conjunctivitis. The same thing has happened before. What is it?**

**Periodic**
**Fever**
**Aphthous stomatitis**
**Pharyngitis**
**Adenitis (cervical)**

**Abbreviated PFAPA**

What is the natural course of PFAPA?

It is benign, but recurrent and annoying

How can you get rid of PFAPA?

Tonsillectomy appears to cure it in most patients!

Prednisone taken at the onset of the episode knocks it out – but may increase recurrences

**Following an injury to an extremity, a child develops long-term pain in the extremity, and intermittent vasomotor changes. The pain is brought on by routine stimuli to the skin. What is the diagnosis?**

**Reflex sympathetic dystrophy**
**(also known as a "chronic regional pain syndrome")**

| | |
|---|---|
| **How can you treat chronic regional pain syndromes?** | PT, psychological support, & neurological pain meds such as amitryptyline |
| **What interventions have been shown to improve symptoms significantly in patients with fibromyalgia?** | Improved sleep<br><br>&<br><br>Exercise |
| Amyloid is sometimes deposited in organs, in association with rheumatologic diseases. How can amyloid deposition be prevented? | Aggressive treatment reduces or eliminates amyloid deposition (especially in the kidney) |
| Is reactive arthritis more common in certain HLA types? | Yes – HLA-B27 |
| If a patient is described who "can't see, can't pee, and can't climb a tree," but the question also describes an unusual rash on the palms, soles, and penis what disorder are you dealing with? | Still reactive arthritis (The rash just doesn't get as much attention! Palm & sole rash by itself is syphilis, though!) |
| If a woman develops reactive arthritis, how will her symptoms be different from those of a man with reactive arthritis? | Women develop cervicitis rather than urethritis (less noticeable, underdiagnosed) |
| Behcet's syndrome causes ocular symptoms and mucocutaneous lesions. How is it different from reactive arthritis? | In Behcet's *small vessel vasculitis* is the problem, affecting multiple organs –<br><br>skin & retinal scarring due to uveitis can occur, myositis & myocarditis are also possible<br><br>*Arthritis is uncommon in Behcet's* |
| **Is Behcet's syndrome more common in certain HLA types?** | **Yes – HLA-B51** |
| Other than the obvious trauma, what other causes of monoarticular arthritis are important? | 1. *Gonorrhea* (especially with onset just after menses)<br>2. Septic joint (not GC)<br>3. Gout & pseudogout (rare in kids) |

| | |
|---|---|
| When examining a patient with monoarticular arthritis, which diagnosis is most worrisome? | Septic joint (any pathogen) |
| Needle-like crystals in joint fluid indicate what diagnosis? | Gout |
| **What is the most common organism, overall, for septic arthritis?** | **Staph aureus** |
| What unusual locations often develop septic arthritis in IV drug users? | Axial skeletal (meaning the ribs, sternum, vertebra, etc.) |
| Joint fluid should have a WBC count how high, in order to be considered a likely septic joint? | >50,000 |
| Is it common to have >75 % PMNs in synovial fluid affected by an inflammatory process? | Yes |
| How can you remember which crystals are positively vs. negatively birefringent in gout & pseudogout? | <u>P</u>seudogout <u>P</u>ositive<br>Needle-like <u>Ne</u>Gative <u>G</u>out |
| **Sickle cell patients are well-known for developing septic arthritis due to which organism?** | **Salmonella** |
| **Staph aureus is the most common cause of septic arthritis in children. Which more unusual pathogens are also likely to cause septic arthritis in infants and very young children?** | **Young infant (<2 months) – E. coli, Group B Strep, and other gram negative bacilli**<br><br>**Young children (2 months to 5 years old) – Group A Strep & Strep pneumoniae** |
| For an acute episode of gout, how would you treat the patient? | NSAIDs<br>Colchicine<br>Systemic or intraarticular steroids |

| | |
|---|---|
| Should a gout patient have a fever? | Often, yes |
| How does gout develop? | Long-term elevation of uric acid |
| Overproduction of uric acid is an *uncommon* reason for developing gout. In what situations does it occur? | Lymphoproliferative/ myeloproliferative disorders (sometimes, not always) |
| What is the usual pathophysiology of gout? | Inadequate *excretion* of uric acid |
| What are three common reasons for impaired uric acid excretion? | 1. Renal insufficiency<br>2. Loop diuretics<br>3. Alcohol |
| Does gout occur in the upper extremities? | Very rarely<br><br>(pseudogout does) |
| **Which gender most often develops gonococcal arthritis?** | **Females** |
| In addition to joints, gonococcus also affects what other connective tissue structure? | Tendons (tendonitis) |
| **Although only one joint is usually affected at a time in gonococcal arthritis, this arthritis often shows what pattern over time?** | **Migratory** |
| **When do the symptoms of gonococcal arthritis usually begin?** | **During or just after menses** |
| **Which tick-borne infectious disease is famous for producing arthritis/arthralgia?** | **Lyme disease** |
| **In addition to joints, what other body systems may Lyme disease affect?**<br>    **(3)** | **1. Skin (erythema migrans rash)**<br>**2. Neurological (facial palsy, headache, neuritis)**<br>**3. Cardiac (heart block & dysrhythmia)** |

Which autoimmune disease is especially common in young, African American, females?

Lupus

(systemic lupus erythematosus or SLE)

**In addition to affecting joints, tendons, and muscles, which other body systems does lupus usually affect?**

1. **Skin (malar rash)**
2. **Renal (nephritis, nephrotic syndrome, and renal failure)**
3. **Neurological (cerebritis, headache, stroke, etc.)**

**What serious cardiac complication sometimes occurs in lupus?**

**Tamponade**

(also causes pericarditis & myocarditis)

What serious GI complication goes with lupus?

Intestinal vasculitis

(can lead to perforation, gangrene, ulcerations, etc.)

Although lupus patients are more likely to clot than average, what (unexpected) hematologic problems are they likely to have?
(2)

1. Anemia
2. Thrombocytopenia

**What is the buzzword for ankylosing spondylitis on X-ray?**

**"Bamboo spine"**

**(looks like a single stick of bamboo)**

**What joint (other than those in the spine) is classically affected in ankylosing spondylitis?**

**Sacroiliac joints**

How is ankylosing spondylitis treated?

Exercise
NSAIDs
Sulfasalazine
Anti-TNF agents

**What two GI disorders are most closely linked to recurrent arthritis?**

**UC & Crohn's**

Uveitis, urethritis, conjunctivitis, and arthritis are the classic presentation of what disorder?

Reactive arthritis

(Can't see,
Can't pee,
Can't climb a tree)

| | |
|---|---|
| Both reactive arthritis and ankylosing spondylitis are usually seen in patients with which HLA type? | B27 |
| Reactive arthritis is usually seen in what type of patient? | Male, 15–35 years old |
| How is a bout of reactive arthritis usually set off, in general terms? | An infection – Usually GI or urethral/cervical |
| How is reactive arthritis treated? | • Treat underlying infection<br>• NSAIDs<br>• Steroids, if needed |
| In addition to conjunctivitis, what other eye problems do reactive arthritis patients often have? | Iritis/uveitis |
| What specific infection is most often linked to reactive arthritis in adolescent & adult populations? | Chlamydial urethritis |
| **Why might a patient with hemophilia have joint inflammation?** | **Due to frequent intraarticular bleeds** |
| **If a patient has small joint arthritis (dactylitis), chronic skin lesions, and is rheumatoid factor negative, what is the likely diagnosis?** | **Psoriasis, with psoriatic arthritis** |
| **How is psoriatic arthritis treated?** | **NSAIDs**<br>**Methotrexate or sulfasalazine**<br>**TNF inhibitors**<br>**(& steroids, if needed)** |
| **How is Lyme disease treated?** | **Amoxicillin**<br><br>**Or**<br><br>**Doxycycline** |
| In pregnant women, how could Lyme disease be treated? | Amoxicillin |

| | |
|---|---|
| **What joint problem do sickle cell patients often suffer from?** | **Avascular necrosis of the femoral head** |
| **Why should you do blood cultures in a septic arthritis patient?** | **The infection usually has a hematogenous source** |
| How is gout or pseudogout treated, in an acute attack? | NSAIDs<br><br>Or<br><br>Colchicine<br>(*microtubule inhibitor – very poorly tolerated*) |
| What two medications can be used for long-term prevention of gout attacks? | Probenicid<br><br>&<br><br>Allopurinol |
| Which gout medication can actually worsen an acute attack of gout? | Allopurinol<br>(may transiently raise the uric acid level) |
| **Rheumatic fever causes a type of arthritis. Which type?** | **Migratory polyarthritis** |
| **Is rheumatic fever an infectious disease?** | No –<br>It's autoimmune |
| **How is rheumatic fever triggered?** | 1. **Genetically predisposed person**<br>2. **Group A β-hemolytic strep infection** |
| **After a strep infection, when will rheumatic fever develop?** | 2–6 weeks later<br><br>(sources vary) |
| **What are the major criteria for rheumatic fever?**<br>(5) | 1. **Carditis**<br>2. **Cutaneous nodules**<br>3. **Chorea**<br>4. **Arthritis**<br>5. **Rash** |
| **How many major criteria for rheumatic fever are needed for the diagnosis?** | Two<br>(or one major & two minor) |

| | |
|---|---|
| **In osteoarthritis, will the joint be red or hot?** | <u>No!</u> |
| **When osteoarthritis affects a joint, what bony malformation is often seen?** | **Bony spurs** |
| When osteoarthritis affects the hands, what is the usual appearance? | Large DIP & PIP joints – *No misalignment* |
| **Patients with rheumatoid arthritis have their worst symptoms during what part of the day?** | **Morning** |
| **Osteoarthritis patients have their worst symptoms in what situation?** | **After using the joint** |
| Will children with rheumatoid arthritis be rheumatoid factor positive? | Usually not |
| **What systemic signs of disease would you expect in a rheumatoid arthritis patient?** | **Fever** <br> & <br> **Malaise** |
| **What skin findings are often seen in rheumatoid arthritis patients?** | **Subcutaneous nodules** |
| **Rheumatoid arthritis often causes changes in the fingers. What are the buzzwords for the finger findings?** (**3**) | 1. **Swan-neck deformity** <br> 2. **Boutonniere deformity** <br> 3. *Ulnar deviation* |
| **How will a joint damaged by rheumatoid arthritis appear on X-ray?** | **Like granulation tissue** <br><br> (Looks like a big fluffy area due to inflammatory changes) |

| | |
|---|---|
| **What is the buzzword for the X-ray appearance of a rheumatoid joint?** | A "pannus"<br><br>(describes the appearance of the fluffy, inflamed cartilage) |
| **What is Legg-Calve-Perthe disease?** | Avascular necrosis of the femoral head |
| **What is Sjogren's syndrome?** | **Dry eyes (keratoconjunctivitis)**<br><br>&<br><br>**Dry mouth (xerostomia)**<br><br>**(often occurs with other autoimmune diseases)** |
| **How are the symptoms of Sjogren's treated?** | **Wetting eye drops**<br><br>&<br><br>**Good oral hygiene**<br><br>**(minimizes symptoms)** |
| **The ANA titer can be used as a screening test for what two common autoimmune disorders?** | *Lupus*<br><br>&<br><br>**Scleroderma** |
| **What lab test confirms the lupus diagnosis?** | **Anti-Smith antibodies** |
| **How is lupus treated?** | **NSAIDs**<br>**Hydroxychloroquine**<br>**Steroids**<br>**Immunomodulators (e.g., azathioprine, cyclophosphamide, methotrexate, mycophenolate)** |
| **What neuropsychiatric problems are sometimes a part of lupus?** | **1. Depression**<br>**2. Seizures**<br>**3. Psychosis** |
| **Which body systems does lupus most often affect?** | **1. Skin**<br>**2. Kidney**<br>**3. Arthritis/joints** |

**Which problem sometimes seen with lupus can lead to sudden death?**

**Pericarditis**

**(Rapid development of an effusion causes the sudden decompensation)**

**What infectious disease assay is often falsely positive in lupus patients?**

**VDRL**
**(syphilis)**

**A positive anticentromere antibody test indicates what connective tissue disease?**

**CREST**

Mnemonic:
Think "antiCRESTomere antibody," and you'll get it right!!

Which disorder is CREST most closely related to?

Scleroderma

What are the problems of the CREST syndrome?

C calcinosis
R Raynaud's phenomenon
E Esophageal dysmotility
S sclerodactyly
T telangiectasia

**Which lab test confirms the scleroderma diagnosis?**

**Antitopoisomerase**

**Mnemonic: A scleroderma diagnosis makes you feel "anti" of being on "top."**

In general, how is scleroderma or CREST treated?

Nothing is very effective
(sorry, trick question)

**Which connective tissue disorder can occasionally present as "heartburn?"**

**Scleroderma**
(The LES loses its effectiveness as it is infiltrated → reflux)

**The most noticeable effect of scleroderma is _____?**

**Thickened skin**
(Noted as decreased wrinkles, taut or shiny skin, limited facial expressions)

**The skin thickening typical of CREST and scleroderma is often noticed first on what part of the body?**

**Hands**

Who is usually afflicted by Behcet's syndrome?

Young adult males

**What are the main complaints seen with Behcet's syndrome?**

<u>Painful</u> oral & genital ulcers

What other rheumatologic complaints often accompany Behcet's syndrome?

Uveitis
Arthralgia
Rashes/lesions
(especially erythema nodosum)

**Which body systems does GPA mainly affect?**

**The respiratory tree, including the nose with nose bleeds & nasal perforations**

**+**

**Kidneys**

**How is GPA treated?**
   **(2)**

1. **Steroids**
2. **Rituximab**
3. **Cyclophosphamide**

**What lab test identifies GPA patients?**

c-ANCA
(an antibody test)

Mnemonic:
Think of an "anchor" (ANCA) shaped like a "wedge" (Weg) dropping in the lung.

**How do GPA patients most often present?**

**Nosebleeds**

   **Or**

**Hemoptysis**

Does GPA cause acute renal failure?

Yes –
& hematuria, of course

**How is dermatomyositis different from polymyositis?**

**The skin is involved**

**What is the most typical skin finding of dermatomyositis?**

**Heliotrope rash**

(purplish rash & edema around the eyes)

**What skin finding is pathognomonic of dermatomyositis, when present?**

**Gottron papules**

(Round, smooth, flat, purple-light red slightly raised areas of the knuckles or along the sides of the fingers)

| | |
|---|---|
| How is dermatomyositis diagnosed? | Muscle biopsy<br><br>Or<br><br>MRI (changes in muscle noted on T2 images) |
| **What patient group most often develops "fibromyalgia?"** | **Young adult females** |
| **How is fibromyalgia diagnosed?** | **By exclusion**<br>**(No abnormal findings)** |
| **What do fibromyalgia patients complain of?** | **Pain throughout the body**<br>**Headaches & dizziness**<br>**Fatigue**<br>**Anxiety/stress**<br>**Insomnia** |
| How is fibromyalgia treated? | Regular schedule<br>Rest & improved sleep quality<br>Aerobic exercise<br>NSAIDs & TCAs (sometimes)<br>A variety of other medications including gabapentin or pregabalin |
| **What kind of disorder is polyarteritis nodosa?** | **A vasculitis** |
| **Which vessels are affected in polyarteritis nodosa?** | **The medium-sized vessels** |
| **What do patients complain of with polyarteritis nodosa?**<br>**(4)** | 1. **Abdominal pain**<br>2. **Weight loss**<br>3. **Kidney problems**<br>4. **Peripheral neuropathy** |
| **What virus is associated with the development of polyarteritis nodosa?** | **Hepatitis B** |
| What will the UA of a polyarteritis patient usually show? | Protein & blood<br>(leaky tubules) |
| Do polyarteritis patients have fever with their disorder? | Yes, often |

**What vasculitis affects mainly Asian women, and involves the aortic arch and its branches?**

**Takayasu arteritis**

**What is the informal name for Takayasu's arteritis? (helps you remember what the disorder is)**

**"Pulseless disease"**

(The vasculitis in various aortic root branches sometimes makes it impossible to get a pulse)

**What patient group is usually affected by Takayasu's arteritis?**

**Young Asian women (15–30 years old)**

How is Takayasu's usually diagnosed?

Characteristic lesions on angiogram

What bad complications are seen regularly with Takayasu's arteritis?
    (2)

1. Stroke (carotid involvement)
2. Heart failure (coronary artery involvement)

**A child who suffers a myocardial infarction has what rheumatological disorder, until proven otherwise?**

**Kawasaki's**

**Kawasaki patients sometimes have arthritis. What type of vessel problems do they develop?**

**Coronary vessel vasculitis, and sometimes dilatation & aneurysms**

**What are the main signs of Kawasaki syndrome?**
    **(6)**

1. **High fever >5 days**
2. **(Truncal) rash**
3. **Strawberry tongue or red, chapped lips**
4. **Conjunctivitis (but no discharge)**
5. **Cervical LAD**
6. **Extremity signs (swelling or erythema)**

**Late in the progression of Kawasaki's, what do you expect to observe with regard to the skin?**

**Desquamation of palms & soles** (peeling)

| | |
|---|---|
| Which kids are most likely to develop Kawasaki's? (3 characteristics) | Asian (especially Japanese & Korean descent) Male <5 years old |
| **How is Kawasaki syndrome treated?** | **Aspirin & IVIG** **(reduces risk of coronary aneurysms)** |
| **Is erythema nodosum a good or bad prognostic for a patient with sarcoid?** | **Good** (It is usually a good sign, in general) |
| **On exam, you notice some flat, smooth, red, areas over the knuckles of a patient who was brought in for fatigue and weakness. What other skin finding is likely in this patient?** | **Heliotrope rash – Probably dermatomyositis** **(The finger findings are Gottron's papules – *very popular photo item!!!*)** |
| **Which CT disorder is associated with anti-dsDNA antibodies?** | **SLE** |
| **Which CT disorder sometimes has anti-Jo-1 antibodies?** | **Polymyositis/dermatomyositis** |
| Which CT disease sometimes has anti-centromere antibodies? | Limited scleroderma (CREST variant – Remember "antiCRESTomere antibody!") |
| Rheumatoid factor goes with _____? | Rheumatoid arthritis (JIA), but mainly in adults |
| **The screening test for SLE is _____?** | **ANA** **(antinuclear antibody)** |
| **Two confirmatory tests for SLE are _____ & _____?** | **Anti-dsDNA antibody** **(double stranded DNA)** & **Anti-Smith antibody** |
| SLE patients are often false positive for what sexually transmitted disease tests? | VDRL/RPR (syphilis – they will be negative for treponeme-specific tests) |

| | |
|---|---|
| **Which molecule predisposes lupus patient to easy clotting/ thrombosis?** | **Antiphospholipid antibody**<br><br>**(Formerly known as lupus anticoagulant – such a bad name!)** |
| **Antineutrophilic cytoplasmic antibody (ANCA) is often positive in which autoimmune disorder?** | **GPA** |
| **A patient positive for both ANA (screening test) and antitopoisomerase (specific test) probably has which disorder?** | **Diffuse scleroderma** |
| A patient positive for both ANA (screening test) and anticentromere antibody (specific test) probably has which disorder? | CREST<br>(limited scleroderma variant) |
| **Antiglomerular antibodies go with which autoimmune disorder?** | **Goodpasture's** |
| **Anti-histone antibody is positive in which autoimmune-related diagnosis?** | <u>Drug-induced</u> lupus |
| What does C-reactive protein tell you in the context of autoimmune disease? | Not much –<br>It's very nonspecific |
| **HLA-B51 goes with which autoimmune disorder?** | **Behcet's** |
| **Anticardiolipin antibodies are often positive in which rheumatological disorder?** | **Lupus**<br>(They are probably responsible for the false positive VDRL, by the way) |
| **Which rheumatological disorder is most associated with antiphospholipid antibodies?** | **Lupus**<br><br>(This antibody is probably related to the thrombophilia) |

| | |
|---|---|
| Which rheumatological disorders are associated with HLA-B27? | Reactive arthritis<br>Ankylosing spondylitis<br>Psoriatic arthritis<br>Enthesitis-related arthritis |
| Diffuse scleroderma patients are often positive for which specific antibody? | Anti-DNA-topoisomerase<br>(aka Scl-70) |
| Antiphospholipid & anticardiolipin antibodies are consistent with which rheumatological disorder? | SLE |
| **SLE patients often are positive for anti-Smith antibody. What is this antibody?** | **Antibody against ribonucleic proteins (RNA)** |
| **Anti-Ro and Anti-La antibodies go with which connective tissue disorder?** | **Sjogren's syndrome<br>(dry eyes, dry mouth)** |
| Polymyositis & dermatomyositis patients often have what specific antibody? | Anti-Jo-1<br>(only 25 % have it, though) |
| **Elevated CK and aldolase are seen in what autoimmune disorder?** | **Polymyositis<br>&<br>Dermatomyositis** |
| **Weakness in proximal muscles, and a heliotrope rash (purple sunrise shape over the eyes) suggest what diagnosis?** | **Dermatomyositis** |
| In addition to Rheumatoid Arthritis, which other connective tissue disorder is often rheumatoid factor positive? | Sjogren's<br>(Joints are usually not affected in Sjogren's) |
| **Which drug is *best known* for causing drug-induced lupus?** | **Hydralazine<br>(also procainamide & isoniazid)** |

**If a drug induces lupus, what happens when the drug is discontinued?**

**It usually goes away**

(The marker for drug-induced lupus is anti-histone antibody, remember)

**In addition to rheumatoid factor, which other antibody test are likely to be positive in Sjogren's syndrome?**

**Anti-Ro**
**Anti-La**

**(aka SS-A & SS-B)**

What is the name for antibodies to ribonucleic proteins?

Anti-Smith antibodies
(lupus)

Diffuse vasculitis with "fibrinoid deposits" affecting arterioles and small arteries =

Systemic lupus erythematosus
(SLE)

**Which type of lupus is often ANA negative???**

**"Discoid" lupus**

**How is discoid lupus different from regular SLE?**

**Only the lesioned skin is affected – no other SLE problems**

What is found in the affected skin of a discoid lupus patient?

Ig-complement complexes

What is the probability of developing SLE, if you already have discoid lupus?

5–10 %

**What special, not life-threatening, heart problem is associated with lupus?**

**Libman-Sacks endocarditis**
**(_not_ infectious)**

**Which valves are affected in Libman-Sacks endocarditis?**

**Mitral**

    **&**

**Tricuspid**

**(the slower flow valves – flow during diastole)**

How are the lesions of Libman-Sacks endocarditis described?

Verrucous (wart-like) –
With fibrinous
& inflammatory components

**Which connective tissue disorder puts you at increased risk of developing lymphoma?**

**Sjogren's**

(10 % or less, though)

**Which is more benign, CREST or scleroderma?**

**CREST**

Anti-Jo-1 antibodies go with which disorder?

Polymyositis

&

Dermatomyositis

# Chapter 8
# Selected Neurology Topics

## Chiari Malformation, Arnold-Chiari Malformation and Dandy-Walker Syndrome

*"Please compare and contrast the following . . ."*

## Chiari & Arnold-Chiari Malformation

*(Evidently, Chiari created the initial classification for types 1–3, so many sources have changed over to just calling them the Chiari malformations. Arnold-Chiari malformation specifically refers to type 2, which Dr. Arnold further described.)*

**Main Ideas**
At minimum, the cerebellar tonsils are below the foramen magnum. On a drawing or radiological image, it looks like the bottom of the cerebellum sort of slid down into the spinal canal by accident.
(You will recall that it is usually a good idea to keep the brain inside the skull!)

Chiari malformation *is **rarely** associated with malformations in other organs.*
Chiari malformation *is **very often** associated with abnormalities of the spinal cord (especially syringomyelia – a fluid-filled & sometimes expanding space in the cord).*

Physical exam may show a *myelomeningocele or occipital encephalocele.*

Brain stem functions can be compromised (life threatening!)

© Springer Science+Business Media New York 2015
C.M. Houser, *Pediatric Tricky Topics, Volume 1*,
DOI 10.1007/978-1-4939-1859-1_8

**Specifics**

There are three main versions of Chiari malformation, with varying degrees of severity. Type 1 is not too bad – only the cerebellar tonsils have come through the foramen magnum.

Types 2 & 3 are worse – In type 2, more of the cerebellum has slid into the spinal canal, and the medulla is displaced downward, also, although in some cases it is still above the foramen magnum. Often, a myelomeningocele (that's when part of the contents of the spinal cord are on the outside of the body, covered by meninges) is also present & partial or complete paralysis occurs below the level of the myelomeningocele.

In type 3, the displacement is severe & the parts that slid down are also outside of the skull or spinal canal, in an encephalocele. It is the most severe and least common of the three main malformations.

Type 2 is classically referred to as "Arnold-Chiari" malformation.


Newly Added

Type 4 is a recent addition – It is cerebellar hypoplasia. The cerebellum is underdeveloped or fails to completely develop. The pathogenesis of type 4 is probably *not* related to the other types of Chiari malformation. Both types 3 & 4 are usually not compatible with life.

Type 0 (zero) may be added – it is currently a matter of debate. In type 0, the patient has typical Chiari malformation-type symptoms, but no detectable anatomical changes.


**Presentation**

Type 1 is often asymptomatic or sometimes doesn't present until adulthood. The patients usually develop nystagmus, occipital headaches with straining, ataxia, and eventually spastic paresis (weakness) in one or more extremities.

Types 2 and 3 usually present in infancy with cranial nerve palsies (swallowing difficulties and stridor) and respiratory difficulties – due to the unusual pressure on the medulla which contains the "breathing center" of the brain. Paralysis below the level of the myelomeningocele is also common.

Due to the malformations involved, the malformation is very often diagnosed before birth, and if not, is clear at the time of birth. Some patients are affected more severely than others, even within the same type.


**Treatment & Prognosis**

Patient with Chiari malformations often develop hydrocephalus. If the patient has hydrocephalus, then they need a ventriculoperitoneal shunt, as usual. Myelomeningoceles & encephaloceles require surgical interventions.

To address the problems of the malformation itself, a posterior fossa "decompression" is done, meaning that the foramen magnum and arch of the atlas (the first vertebral body) is removed, to provide more space. Despite this intervention, some patients continue to worsen (reason unclear).

Treatment for patients with symptomatic Chiari type 1 malformations generally have positive surgical outcomes, but greater functional deficits prior to surgery often means greater residual deficits after surgery.

### Mnemonic
Think of *Arnold* (Schwarzenegger) in the Terminator movie, and imagine that his cyborg brain has dropped down into the spinal canal a bit, due to a bad fight (types 1 & 2).

When the fight gets *really bad*, his back is ripped open, and he ends up with part of his cyborg spinal cord sticking brain sticking out (type 2), or brain sticking out of his neck (type 3).

## Dandy-Walker Syndrome

### Main Ideas
*The problem is that the foramina (plural of foramen) of Luschka and Magendie don't form properly, and are basically closed.* This means that, for most patients, all of the ventricles enlarge, *especially the fourth ventricle.*

A giant fourth ventricle means that there was pressure on the cerebellum when it was trying to form, so it is very small – just like a lung that tries to develop with gut herniated into the chest cavity during fetal development.

It is *very common* for Dandy-Walker patients to have abnormalities in other body systems (65 %), especially in the cardiac system.

*The problems in other body systems mainly determine their prognosis.*

Physical exam may show a *prominent occiput*.

### Presentation
Prominent occiput, and hydrocephalus (about 80 %).

50 % have intellectual disability (previously known as mental retardation), and as you would expect, most have cerebellar signs – ataxia, poor fine motor coordination, and some spasticity. 15 % have seizures.

**Treatment & Prognosis**

If hydrocephalus is present, the *fourth ventricle* needs to be shunted (not the lateral ventricles, which is the usual place to locate the shunt).

Good prognosis – although cognitive & functional disabilities are likely.

(Problems in other, non-neurological, systems will primarily determine the prognosis.)


**Mnemonic**

It's hard to walk "like a dandy" with no cerebellum!

So . . . in Arnold-Chiari – parts of the brain (cerebellum and medulla) are being squished by the surrounding bone – due to bad positioning of the neural structures. (Mom always told you it wasn't good to slouch!)

In Dandy-Walker – the cerebellum *(but not the brainstem)* is being squished by fluid – due to the bone developing without the usual exits for the CSF.


# Syringomyelia

Syringomyelia is defined as a cavitation (cavity formation) in the spinal cord, filled with fluid, but not normally under pressure. The term came from the Greek word "syrinx" meaning cavity.

In adults, syringomyelia is often a chronic *and progressive* loss of tissue in the spinal cord (although it sometimes occurs in nearby CNS structures). The progress of the disorder is slow. Men are affected more often than women for unknown reasons.

In children, research suggests that many are stable or may even regress. Thus monitoring, & in some cases periodic imaging, is warranted but further intervention often is not.

Idiopathic syringomyelia is thought to be congenital in some cases, but it often doesn't present until the person is in their 20s or 30s due to the slowly progressive nature of the problem. Other cases develop following trauma to the cord (usually blunt) or after infections of the cord, meninges, or other nearby structures. Syringomyelia can develop as a consequence of cord tethering, pressure damage from tumors, or from congenital Chiari malformation and/or hydrocephalus. (Remember that Chiari malformation is the presence of the cerebellar tonsils and medulla in the cervical spinal canal.)

Information regarding the optimal management of idiopathic or incidentally found syringomyelias in pediatric patients is sparse. Serial imaging is usually conducted, to monitor for changes requiring surgical intervention. In many cases, the patient does have symptoms from the lesion, but available data suggest that the symptoms

& symptom severity do not correlate well with the size of the lesion. Idiopathic pediatric syringomyelias often remain stable in size & some spontaneously improve, at least over short follow-up periods of about 2 years.

Syringomyelia is associated with scoliosis. Syringomyelias usually progress down the cord, but in some cases they go up.

The presentation of symptomatic syringomyelia is similar to that of anterior cord syndrome. Initially, patients notice a loss of pain and temperature below level of lesion *with preserved posterior column functions (position sense, two-point discrimination, and deep pressure sensation are intact)*. Motor dysfunction also develops as anterior horn cells are damaged. The motor and sensory problems may be unilateral, bilateral and symmetric, or bilateral and asymmetric.

Diagnosis of syringomyelia is made clinically initially, and then confirmed with MRI (although CT scanning is also possible, MRI is preferred in this situation). Treatments are aimed at reducing the pressure on the cord to arrest progression of the deficits. Treatment is usually surgical.

## Assorted Neuropathology Topics

**Von Hippel-Lindau syndrome** – An autosomal dominant disorder characterized by several types of both benign and malignant neoplasms affecting multiple organs.

1. Bilateral renal cell carcinoma
2. Pheochromocytoma
3. Angiomas of liver, kidney, or other viscera
4. Hemangioblastomas of the retina, cerebellum, & medulla oblongata

The retinal tumors frequently cause visual problems for these patients, and the other hemangioblastomas in the CNS are an important cause of death for these patients.

**Frontal eye fields** – An area of the prefrontal cortex (meaning cortex anterior to the motor strip) that directs visual attention. There is one on each side, and they mainly control saccadic eye movements (with help from the brain stem nuclei) along with causing release of inhibition from the nigral projections to the brain stem. This allows saccades to proceed normally.

*(Saccade means the jumping movement of the eyes from one point of fixation to another – like what your eyes are doing as you read the words printed across the page.)*

Output from each frontal eye field pushes the eyes away from itself. Hyperactivity in this area, such as from a seizure, will cause the gaze to deviate away from the seizure focus. Decreased activity in this area, such as from infarct or trauma, will cause the eyes to deviate toward the lesion – because the only input is now coming from the non-damaged frontal eye field on the other side.

If a patient had bilateral frontal eye field damage (very rare indeed!) it would produce a syndrome in which the patient had no voluntary eye movement at all, but full-range of extraocular movement with random eye movement.

**Medial longitudinal fasciculus (MLF)** – The MLF is mainly important for its role in another acronymic disorder – INO (internuclear ophthalmoplegia). The MLF links the lateral and medial recti nuclei, coordinating horizontal gaze. A lesion in this area therefore produces a dissociation of the two eyes when the patient attempts to gaze to either side. The type of gaze symptom is called "dissociated horizontal nystagmus" because when one eye fails to adduct, the eye behaving normally (abducting) develops nystagmus trying to pull its failing brother over to a conjugate position. The problem can be unilateral or bilateral.

This problem is different from a CN3 nerve or nucleus lesion because the pupil is not affected (and because some limited adduction does occur).

The MLF has a role in vestibulo-ocular reflexes, also.

**Lambert-Eaton syndrome vs. myasthenia gravis** *(note: you may see either Lambert or Eaton written first for this disorder)*

This disorder is sometimes known as *"myasthenic syndrome."* Typically (about 50 % of the time), the disorder is a paraneoplastic syndrome most often associated with small cell lung cancer. Occasionally it occurs in patients without any underlying malignancy. In this disorder, inadequate amounts of ACh are released at neuromuscular junctions producing muscular weakness, decreased deep tendon reflexes, and muscle fatigue. There are two main clinical features that differentiate this syndrome from myasthenia gravis. First, the patient's performance *improves* with increasing activity. Second, the *bulbar muscles are usually not affected.*

Approximately 50 % of Eaton-Lambert syndrome patients also have autonomic dysfunction of the cholinergic system. This means they may experience impotence, dry mouth, and difficulties with vision.

Quick definitions:

Hemihypesthesia – decreased sensation of one-half of the body
Hypesthesia – decreased sensation somewhere
Prosopagnosia – inability to recognize or perceive faces in the absence of any visual system deficit.
Dysprosodia – lack of normal intonation or variation in speech tone, or lack of understanding of the same
Anosmia – inability to smell (usually due to a deceleration injury damaging CN1 where the tufts of the nerve stick through the cribriform plate in the upper nasopharynx)

# Canavan Disease

Canavan disease (aspartoacylase deficiency) is a white matter disease of the brain that occurs due to an autosomal recessive enzyme deficiency.

It is most common in Ashkenazi Jewish populations.

Canavan disease is also known as a "leukodystrophy," which just means white matter deterioration disease. Eventually, the white matter problem turns into overall cerebral atrophy.

*Pathophysiology*:

The specific enzyme deficiency for Canavan disease is aspartoacylase. If you are missing this enzyme, you end up with too much N-acetylaspartic acid (NAA). In patients with aspartoacylase deficiency, NAA is present in many tissues, but it mainly accumulates in the brain and urine. In the brain, it leads to diffuse, symmetrical degeneration of the white matter.

*Presentation and Course*:

The disorder presents as hypotonia, macrocephaly, and head lag between three and six months old. Eventually, they develop hypertonia and hyperreflexia. Blindness from optic atrophy develops between six and eighteen months. Seizures occur in 50 percent of patients. Neurological impairment worsens with time, with bulbar dysfunction developing which leads to feeding difficulties. Spasticity and respiratory complications are also common.

There is no cure for this disease, and management is supportive. Palliative care is essential as death occurs in childhood, usually before 10 years of age, with *very* limited quality of life.

# Chapter 9
# General Neurology Question and Answer Items

| | |
|---|---|
| How common is it to have a single seizure among the general population? | About 5 % |
| **What are the two terms you can use for a seizure affecting just one part of the body?** | **Focal (old term) or Partial (new term)** |
| **What differentiates a "simple" from a "complex" seizure?** | **Simple means no change in level of consciousness**<br><br>**Complex means there was a change** |
| **What is a "generalized" seizure?** | **Seizure affecting both hemispheres from the start** |
| **What does it mean if a seizure is "secondarily generalized?"** | **Started in one location (partial seizure) then spread to both hemispheres** |
| If you see an EEG on the boards, how hard should you work to read it? | Not hard at all – treat the patient, not the EEG |
| **Which type(s) of seizure *does not* have a postictal phase?** | **Absence & Simple Partial** |
| **If the eye fields of the brain are involved in a seizure, do the eyes go toward or away from the seizure?** | **Away (Overactive frontal eye fields push the eyes away)** |

© Springer Science+Business Media New York 2015
C.M. Houser, *Pediatric Tricky Topics, Volume 1*,
DOI 10.1007/978-1-4939-1859-1_9

**If a child is getting into trouble for annoying behaviors or not paying attention, what sort of seizures should you consider?**

**Absence or complex partial**

During a complex partial seizure with automatisms, will the child be able to respond to outside stimuli?

Not normally, but some responsiveness

What is the best way to test for any remaining level of consciousness in an impaired patient?

Painful stimulation

What is the most common sort of automatism to occur in an absence seizure?

Blinking
(but remember that automatisms are most common with complex partial seizures)

What is the best medication for absence seizures?

Ethosuximide

Should Benign Rolandic seizures be treated?

Only if frequent/problematic

What group of patients typically develops Rolandic seizures?

School-aged kids who are otherwise fine

What *is* a benign Rolandic seizure?

A partial seizure that sometimes generalizes – usually occurs at night

Why are they called "Rolandic" seizures?

There is a characteristic spike on EEG over the Rolandic fissure area

What is the other name for benign Rolandic seizures?

Benign childhood epilepsy with CentroTemporal Spikes (BCECTS)

**What is the usual course of benign Rolandic seizures?**

**Spontaneously resolve (by age 15 years)**

**Why is it important to know about benign Rolandic seizures?**

- **Common cause of epilepsy (about 15 % of childhood cases)**
- **No treatment needed**
- **Spontaneous resolution expected**

**The 3-Hz per second spike-and-wave pattern is famous for being associated with what type of seizure?**

**Absence**

What are the two paths patients with absence seizures are likely to follow as they get older?

- Resolution in adolescence
- Epilepsy (30 %)

**Which epilepsy syndrome is known for being induced by visual stimuli?**

**Juvenile myoclonic epilepsy**

**What sort of seizure will the patient have, if he/she has a visually induced seizure?**

**Could be myoclonic only, or could be myoclonic with absence or tonic-clonic**

How do you treat visually induced myoclonic seizures?

Avoid the stimuli (or wear dark glasses, if needed)

"Incoordination" or jerking movements in the early morning are sometimes the first signs of which seizure disorder?

Juvenile myoclonic epilepsy

What do infantile spasms look like?

Spasms of the flexors – especially head & trunk

**What is the special buzzword associated with the EEG appearance of infantile spasms?**

**"Hypsarrhythmia"**

What does hypsarrhythmia mean?

The EEG has a slow rhythm, and is disorganized

*(Specifically – very high voltage, random, slow waves and spikes in all cortical areas)*

Which genetic disorder is especially associated with infantile spasms?

Tuberous sclerosis
(although lots of others cause it, too)

Which type of pediatric seizure has the worst prognosis?

Infantile spasm

What proportion of children with infantile spasm will go on to have epilepsy?

Around 60 %

When children with infantile spasms later develop epilepsy, which type of epilepsy often evolves?

Lennox-Gastaut syndrome (difficult to control, multiple types of seizures associated with intellectual disability)

*Note: The term "mental retardation" while most familiar to many medical practitioners, has now been replaced by the term "intellectual disability" in many sources. Mental retardation has also been eliminated as a term in the 2013 revision of the Diagnostic & Statistical Manual of Mental Disorders, and in US federal legislation.*
*In 2015, however, the ICD-11 international classification of diseases will adopt the term "intellectual developmental disorder" to replace both the terms "mental retardation" & "intellectual disability." This term will then replace intellectual disability in many sources.*

**What is the main danger in treating seizure disorders?**

**Respiratory arrest – (more patients die of medication complications than die of seizures!)**

**If a child has had a febrile seizure, is there risk of developing epilepsy increased?**

**Yes – it's doubled, *but* still very small (0.5 vs. 1.0 – exact numbers quoted vary, some recent studies suggest it might be as high as 2.4)**

The number traditionally quoted, and most likely to occur on exams, is the doubling to 1 %.

If you think you have a child with breath holding spells, what can reassure you that it is, in fact, breath holding?

The sequence –
Pain/anger/fear →
Crying →
Breath holding

If a child has jerking movements after losing consciousness, does that make it less likely that the episode was really a breath holding spell?

No – the child may jerk, be limp, or stiff after losing consciousness

Children with breath holding spells have a higher than average likelihood of also having what physiological disorder?

Anemia/iron deficiency

Why do Klippel-Feil patients have limited neck motion?

Some or all of their cervical vertebra are fused

**What is the "triad" of Klippel-Feil syndrome?**

**Short neck**
**Limited neck motion**
**Low occipital hairline**
**(all neck related!)**

Risk for serious neurological problems in Klippel-Feil patients is highest if the fusion occurs in what part of the c-spine?

Occipito-C1 vertebral junction

Is it common for Klippel-Feil patients to have associated anomalies?

Yes

**What is lissencephaly?**

**Smooth brain (gyri are missing)**

With which congenital syndrome is lissencephaly most associated?

Miller-Dieker

**What is schizencephaly?**

**Clefts in the cerebral hemispheres that weren't supposed to be there**

**(remember "schizo" means split, so schizencephaly is extra "splits" of the brain)**

What sorts of clinical problems does schizencephaly create, if any?

Seizures, severe intellectual disability, quadriparesis

**What is porencephaly?**

**Holes (pores) within the brain**

How would a child develop porencephaly?
  (2 ways)

Usually occurs due to damage from stroke or infection after birth

Can also be congenital, due to developmental error(s)

What is acquired porencephaly?

*(formerly called pseudoporencephaly!)*

Special name for acquired holes in the brain, not due to developmental processes

How can pseudoporencephaly be distinguished from congenital porencephaly?

Congenital porencephalic cysts communicate with the ventricle or subarachnoid space, acquired cysts generally do not

&

Acquired porencephaly is not associated with other CNS malformations

How will acquired porencephaly patients present?

Focal findings, seizures, or sometimes asymptomatic

Do congenital porencephaly patients present differently from acquired porencephaly?

Congenital patients often have more global problems, such as intellectual disability, cerebral palsy, and blindness

If you're born without a corpus callosum, what sorts of problems should you expect to experience?

Some neuropsychiatric difficulties, but often subtle

(75 % of these patients have normal intelligence & otherwise normal appearing function)

**Why would someone fail to develop a corpus callosum?**

1. **Inherited – both AD and AR**
2. **In utero injury prior to the 20th week of pregnancy**
3. **Association to some in utero exposures, especially alcohol**

Holoprosencephaly is highly associated with what very unusual facial abnormality?

Cyclopia (single eye)

What is the most severe form of holoprosencephaly?

"Alobar"
(this means that no lobes formed in the front part of the brain at all)

| | |
|---|---|
| What is the most obvious structural finding if you scan a patient with alobar holoprosencephaly? | Single ventricle |
| How long do alobar holoprosencephaly patients usually survive? | A few months |
| **Use of which recreational drug are associated with agenesis of the corpus callosum?** | **Alcohol & cocaine** |
| **What is static encephalopathy?** | **Cerebral dysfunction that doesn't *worsen* over time (it's allowed to improve)** |
| If a patient is encephalopathic due to high ammonia levels, would that be considered static encephalopathy? | No – whatever caused the encephalopathy must be a completed process leaving changed cerebral function to use this label |
| **What type of problem does the term "cerebral palsy" refer to?** | **Motor** |
| Technically, what is a convulsion? | A seizure due to a cortical lesion (most seizures have this mechanism) |
| Is cerebral palsy a type of static encephalopathy? | Yes – motor only |
| What aspects of motor function can cerebral palsy affect? | Posture, tone, & movement (of course) |
| **Do the problems that cause cerebral palsy occur during, before, or just after birth?** | **Any of those (often the timing of the event is not clear)** |
| **Are sensory problems a part of cerebral palsy?** | **No** |
| **Is perinatal asphyxia the major causal factor in development of cerebral palsy?** | **No** (<10 % of cases are thought to be related to perinatal asphyxia) |

What is the perinatal asphyxia-related factor that gives a high likelihood of later CP?

Metabolic acidosis
(umbilical artery pH < 7 and base deficit > 12 at time of delivery)

What are three known risk factors for the development of CP?

Prematurity/low birth weight
Intrauterine infection
Congenital malformations

Is low birth weight associated with CP?

Yes
(but the causal relationship is not clear)

Low birth weight is especially associated with what sort of CP?

Spastic diplegia
(mainly affects the legs, but arms can be involved too)

Infection is most associated with what sort of CP?

Spastic quadriplegia
(all four extremities are affected)

Which aspects of the immune system have been implicated in CP?

Immune mediators, e.g., interleukins, interferons, and TNF factors

(higher than normal levels may disrupt developing neural circuitry)

What does "spastic CP" mean?

Same types of findings as upper motor neuron lesions – hypertonic & hyperreflexic, clonus, & weakness

What are the subtypes of spastic CP?

Hemiplegia (one side)
Quadriplegia (both sides – all four extremities)
Diplegia (both sides, but legs more affected than arms or face)

Dyskinetic CP is another type of CP. What is its presentation?

Purposeless movements that disappear during sleep – often choreoathetoid and dystonic movements
(truncal twisting, grimacing, etc.)

What is the underlying problem in dyskinetic CP?

Abnormal basal ganglia

Is it possible to have both dyskinetic and spastic CP?

Yes, unfortunately

| | |
|---|---|
| **Which sort of CP has the fewest associated problems?** | **Dyskinetic** |
| **Which children with CP are most likely to have intellectual disability?** <br> **(2 types of CP)** | **Mixed (meaning spastic & non-spastic types of CP in the same person)** <br> & <br> **Spastic quadriplegic** |
| **Is intellectual disability common among kids with CP?** | **Yes – about 50 %** |
| **Which types of CP are most associated with seizure disorder?** | **Spastic hemiplegia & quadriplegia** |
| **Has botulinum toxin been used successfully in spastic CP?** | **Yes – for focal problem areas of spasm** |
| **What relatively new treatment, involving a muscle relaxant, has been shown to be helpful in spastic CP?** | **Intrathecal baclofen** |
| **What oral meds are used to decrease the spasticity in CP?** | **Baclofen** <br> **Dantrolene** <br> **Benzodiazepines (diazepam, clonazepam)** |
| If an infant had a stroke in utero, how will that child present (assuming it is detected clinically)? | Hemiplegic CP *or early hand dominance* |
| **Complications from congenital heart disease account for what proportion of strokes in children?** | 1/4 |
| When is the most dangerous time for a child with congenital heart disease, in terms of stroke risk? | Cardiac cath or surgery – <br> 1/2 of the strokes happen within 3 days of one of these |
| **How important are pro-thrombotic factors in childhood strokes?** | **Important – 1/3 to 1/2 of children who stroke have them** |

**If a child has antiphospholipid antibody, what will he/she be predisposed to develop?**

**Clots – including stroke**

What does lupus anticoagulant put the patient at risk for?

Clotting (it was a poor name choice)

Which types of antiphospholipid antibodies are most commonly implicated in childhood stroke?

Anticardiolipin antibody & lupus anticoagulant
(these are both types of antiphospholipid antibodies)

Which other prothrombotic factors are known to be important contributors to stroke in children and young adults?
   (5)

Protein C
Protein S
Antithrombin III
Elevated homocysteine
Factor 5 Leiden

If a child has a stroke between birth and age two, what are the two most common presentations?

Seizure or hemiplegia

If a child presents with an apparent hemiplegia, what two other diagnoses should you consider in addition to structural damage to the brain?

Complicated migraine

&

Todd's paralysis
(following a seizure)

What bizarre possibility should you consider when a child suddenly develops hemiplegia and no cause can be found?

"alternating hemiplegia"

(Very rare disorder with hemiplegia that switches sides, and seizures between episodes of hemiplegia. Course is progressive neuro deterioration)

What is ataxic CP?

Damage to cerebellum results in coordination & gait problems

**How important is sickle cell disease, as a cause of stroke in children?**

**Important – $\geq 10$ %**

In what age range is stroke most common for SC kids?

2–5 years
(rare <2 years)

Higher levels of hemoglobin F are helpful to sickle cell patients, in general. Does it protect the patient from stroke?

No

**Is it common for sickle cell children to have asymptomatic strokes?**

**Yes – 1 in 5**
**(the brain is very adaptable in young children, and if the area is small and/ or non-critical, there may not be any symptoms)**

**Which are more common in children – ischemic strokes or hemorrhagic strokes?**

**Equally common**

Which are more fatal in children – ischemic strokes or hemorrhagic strokes?

Hemorrhagic (>25 %!)

For sickle cell patients, how can you predict which ones are at special risk for stroke?

Transcranial Doppler flow studies – high flow means increased risk

**What is moyamoya disease?**

**It's really a description, not a disease – chronic occlusion of small cerebral vessels causes collaterals to form**

**What is the buzzword for appearance of moyamoya on scans or angiography?**

**"Puff of smoke" – a dense area of wispy vessels is seen**

In children, moyamoya is associated with which disorders? (4)

Sickle cell
Trisomy 21
Neurofibromatosis (type 1)
& Radiation treatment

Stroke symptoms are occasionally caused by another sort of problem, not thrombus, embolus, or hemorrhage. What problem is that?

Arterial dissection – usually of the internal carotid

**What is the most common cause of CNS vasculitis in children?**

**Bacterial meningitis**

| | |
|---|---|
| **What percentage of children who have had bacterial meningitis also have evidence of a CNS infarct?** | **About 10 %** |
| **When chickenpox is associated with stroke, when does the stroke develop?** | **Within 12 months of the rash**<br><br>(recent data suggests the risk may be limited to the first 6 months, but this is still under investigation) |
| **Which kids are most likely to develop chicken pox associated strokes?** | **<10 years old** |
| **Where do infarcts usually occur, when stroke follows chicken pox?** | **Internal capsule or basal ganglia**<br><br>(think of it as subcortical motor stuff) |
| Which two rheumatologic diseases are rare causes of CNS vasculitis in children? | Lupus & Takayasu arteritis (usually seen in Asian females) |
| If a child has a stroke without a clear etiology, what metabolic disorders should you consider? | ↑ homocysteine<br>MELAS disease<br>Fabry disease |
| What is MELAS disease? | Mitochondrial myopathy<br>Encephalopathy<br>Lactic Acidosis<br>Stroke-like episodes |
| Why does Fabry disease predispose children to stroke? | Ceramide builds up in the vascular endothelial cells, narrowing the vessels<br><br>(specifically, it is globotriaosylceramide that builds up)<br><br>(α-galactosidase deficiency) |
| If a child does not have homocystinuria, should you still consider elevated homocysteine as a possible contributor to a stroke? | Yes, if the stroke was ischemic –<br>We have recently learned that many things increase homocysteine levels (meds, cigarettes, renal disease, thyroid disease, vitamin deficiency, etc.) |

| | |
|---|---|
| Why do elevated homocysteine levels lead to stroke, anyway? | High levels damage vascular endothelium, promoting thrombus formation |
| Is neonatal stroke more common in full-term or preterm infants? | Full term |
| **Are neonatal strokes usually embolic or thrombotic?** | **Embolic (the placenta is thought to be the most common source)** |
| | Note: Ischemic & hemorrhagic strokes are equally common in *children* – ischemic stroke is more common in neonates |
| **Which cerebral artery is most often involved in neonatal stroke?** | *Left* **MCA (middle cerebral artery)** |
| What is the *best* diagnostic for finding a stroke in a neonate? | MRI

(Remember, US is *not* going to show you much in an ischemic stroke) |
| **How do neonates with stroke usually present?** | **Seizures** |
| If a neonate seizes as a result of a cerebrovascular accident, is he/she likely to have a long-term seizure disorder? | No – antiseizure medication may be needed for a few months, but usually not long-term |
| In addition to emboli, another common cause of stroke in neonates is _____? | Hypoxic-ischemic insult |
| What do you expect to see in a full-term infant who has hypoxic-ischemic encephalopathy? | Quadriparesis clinically – Parasagittal damage on imaging |
| What do you expect to see in a preemie who has hypoxic-ischemic encephalopathy? | Lower extremity weakness clinically – periventricular leukomalacia on imaging |
| **How does hypoxic-ischemic encephalopathy cause damage to the brain?** | **Multiple mechanisms: Hypoxia & asphyxia Ischemia & acidosis** |

| | |
|---|---|
| **What is the most common cause of intracranial bleeding in children?** | **Trauma** |
| What are the other common reasons for intracranial bleeding in children? | Coagulopathy<br>Vascular malformation<br>Aneurysm |
| **Typical signs of intraparenchymal bleeding are _____?** | **Seizure**<br>**Focal neuro problem**<br>**Headache**<br>**Change in mental status** |
| **Typical signs of subarachnoid bleeding are _____?** | **"Worst headache of my life" & change in mental status** |
| **What is the best diagnostic choice for acute intracranial bleeding in anyone who doesn't have a fontanelle?** | **Head CT**<br>**(no contrast – new blood is bright)** |
| **What is the most common type of intracranial vascular malformation in children?** | **Venous angiomas – usually benign, no treatment needed** |
| Which type(s) of intracranial malformations usually require surgical intervention? | AVMs<br>(some may be embolized, others require surgical removal) |
| **Which disorders are associated with saccular aneurysms?** | **Aortic coarctation**<br>**Ehlers-Danlos**<br>**Marfan's**<br>**Autosomal dominant polycystic kidney disease**<br><br>**(many other disorders also have some association with saccular aneurysms)** |
| What is the other term for saccular aneurysms? | Berry aneurysms |
| Where are berry aneurysms usually found? | Anterior half of the circle of Willis |

Should intracranial aneurysms be routinely removed?

No – it depends on the aneurysm.

(If it becomes symptomatic, it definitely needs to be removed)

The main risk for patients with berry aneurysms is _____?

Subarachnoid hemorrhage

Can a thrombotic event lead to headache, papilledema, nausea, vomiting, and 6th cranial nerve palsy – all without other localizing signs?

Yes – Superior sagittal sinus thrombosis (CSF return to the venous system is blocked)

Proptosis, chemosis, and ophthalmoplegia can result from what thrombotic event?

Cavernous sinus thrombosis (usually related to cavernous sinus infection from nearby facial sinuses)

The sagittal sinus and cavernous sinus are examples of what general type of structure?

Cerebral veins

What are the main risk factors for cerebral vein thrombosis?

Dehydration & Prothrombotic disorders (which are also called "thrombophilias")

What is the most common presentation for a neonate with a cerebral vein thrombosis?

Seizure

What is the most common presentation for children with cerebral vein thrombosis?

Headache with nausea/vomiting

If you are worried about cerebral vein thrombosis, what will a screening head CT usually show?

Often nothing – contrast is usually needed to see the clot

What is the diagnostic test of choice to diagnose cerebral vein thrombosis?

MRI/MRA with contrast

How worried should you be about a patient who has a cerebral vein thrombosis?

Worried – 20 % bad M&M (about 5 % mortality & 15 % with long term sequelae)

| | |
|---|---|
| **An adolescent female is diagnosed with optic neuritis on the board exam. What disorder do you suspect she has/will have?** | **Multiple sclerosis (about 50 % of optic neuritis patients will develop MS)** |
| **Band-like sensory abnormalities, incoordination, oculomotor disturbance, and vision abnormalities are typical presenting symptoms for which disorder?** | **Multiple sclerosis** |
| The best way to diagnose multiple sclerosis is _____? | *Clinically!* It is the only way. |
| **What is the basic clinical criterion for an MS diagnosis?** | **Deficits that vary in time and place (location within the brain)** |
| What imaging test is often helpful in making a multiple sclerosis diagnosis? | MRI – looking for areas of demyelination |
| If you suspect MS, but the patient's MRI is normal, does that rule-out the diagnosis? | No |
| If you've ordered an MRI on a patient with focal neurological abnormalities not consistent with MS, and the MRI report comes back with focal areas c/w MS, does that mean the patient has MS? | No – A small but significant proportion of the normal population has these "spots" on MRI |
| What lab test can be helpful to making an MS diagnosis? | CSF with high IgG or "oligoclonal bands" |
| It is rare to develop MS before what age? | 10 years old |
| Traditional treatment for MS exacerbations relies mainly on what two medications? | Steroids & ACTH |

**What is the most common type of childhood seizure?**

Generalized (60 %)

The buzzwords for the EEG appearance of a generalized seizure are _____ & _____?

Bilateral & synchronous

Do patients with generalized seizures typically have an aura before the seizure?

No – it would be better if they did, so they could go sit down!

Generalized seizures in very young children are often different in presentation from those of older children. How?

Usually tonic *or* clonic, rather than a mix of both

What is the deal with myoclonic seizures – is there a change of consciousness or not?

Depends on length of seizure – very brief ones don't affect mental status. Long ones often do.

What is special about the relationship of myoclonic seizures to other seizure types?

Myoclonic sometimes occurs *with* absence or tonic-clonic seizures

**Myoclonic seizures should classically have what characteristics?**

**Short episode of quick bilateral muscle contractions – may be one or multiple jerks involved**

**Do myoclonic seizures put the patient at risk for falls?**

**Yes**

Patients with myoclonic seizure disorders are more likely than average to also have what sort of chronic diseases?

Neurodegenerative

Which seizure disorder runs in families, and is especially likely to appear with sleep deprivation or alcohol use?

Juvenile myoclonic epilepsy

A sudden loss of muscle tone, with loss of consciousness, sometimes preceded by one or two myoclonic jerks is what type of seizure disorder?

Atonic or akinetic seizure disorder (both names are used)

The common name for these is "drop attacks"

Which children are most likely to develop atonic seizures?

Static encephalopathy/Lennox-Gastaut syndrome kids

What is the treatment for akinetic seizures?

No good one

**A patient of normal intelligence is presented who complains of bilateral jerking movements in the morning. Episodes began in the preteen years. What is the disorder?**

**Juvenile myoclonic epilepsy**

In addition to bilateral involuntary jerking movements in the morning, the patient's girlfriend told him that sometimes he has an all-out seizure in the morning. What disorder is that?

Still juvenile myoclonic epilepsy – some have generalized tonic-clonic morning seizures

Janz syndrome is the other name for which seizure disorder?

Juvenile myoclonic epilepsy (they both start with "J")

What is the drug of choice for treating juvenile myoclonic epilepsy?

Valproate

**What is the main worry in terms of serious side effects with using valproate?**

1. **Hepatotoxicity (especially in preschoolers)**
2. **Pancreatitis**

What are the more common, but less worrisome, side effects of valproate?
      (5)

Nausea or weight gain, hair loss, thrombocytopenia, sleepiness

**Which antiseizure medication can be used with any of the common seizure types?**

**Valproate**

Are absence seizures generalized or focal?

Generalized

**How long does an absence seizure usually last?**

**A few seconds (not more than 10)**

**Are there any movements that often accompany absence seizures?**

No big movements – flickering eyelids are common, though!

What is the old (French) name for absence seizures?

Petit mal

**How can you tell an absence seizure from a complex partial seizure?**

**Absence is:**
**Short (<10 s)**
**No aura**
**No postictal phase**

**Is it possible to induce an absence seizure in children who don't normally have them?**

**Yes, with 3–4 min of hyperventilation (even gives you classic EEG 3 cycles/ second waves)**

Is there a familial form of absence epilepsy, and if so, how is it inherited?

Yes – multifactorial
The children grow out of it in adolescence

**What are simple partial seizures?**

**Seizures that affect only one area of the cortex – usually motor, but can be sensory or cognitive (e.g., hallucinations)**

**What is the most common type of simple partial seizure?**

**Motor**

**How long do simple partial seizures last?**

**Short – 10 to 20 s**

**Do you expect a postictal phase, or aura, with simple partial seizures?**

**No – neither**

**Complex partial seizures usually come from what part of the brain?**

**Limbic system
(names like amygdala, hippocampus, and "mesial" temporal lobe)**

**What is the most common specific anatomic abnormality seen in children with complex partial seizures?**

**Hippocampal sclerosis**

**Is a postictal phase expected with complex partial seizures?**

**Yes**

| | |
|---|---|
| What is the likelihood that a complex partial seizure patient will become seizure free on meds? | <1/3 |
| What are the drugs of choice for complex partial seizures in pediatrics? (2 preferred, and 2 backup) | Carbamazepine & oxcarbazepine Phenytoin & valproate are also appropriate first line agents, but the two above are generally preferred (many antiseizure medication options, and combinations of medications, are possible) |
| Which type of seizure patient is most often a candidate for surgical intervention? | Complex partial (due to poor control with meds) |
| Can someone have an "emotional" seizure? | Yes – *complex* partial temporal lobe seizures can consist mainly of an intense emotional experience |
| What is the other name for infantile spasms? | West syndrome (Think of facing *West* to *salaam*, the position of an infantile spasm – Lennox-Gastaut comes later) |
| Infantile spasms typically occur in what age group? | Less than 12 months old, of course! (that's why they call it infantile) |
| **What does an infantile spasm look like?** | **The politically incorrect way to remember it is as a "salaam" attack – the child suddenly flexes head and trunk** |
| How many spasms usually occur at a time? | Anywhere from several to hundreds |
| What is the eponymic name sometimes used for infantile spasm? | West syndrome |
| Is the DTaP vaccine related to the development of infantile spasms? | No |
| What is the most common treatment for infantile spasms? | ACTH (vigabatrin is also used) |

| | |
|---|---|
| How successful is treatment for infantile spasms? | Not very good |
| **What is the natural course of infantile spasms?** | **Spontaneously resolves by 5 years old, but the children develop severe intellectual disability & other seizure types develop** (Lennox-Gastaut) |
| **What defines Lennox-Gastaut syndrome?** (3 features) | • **Severe & multiple types of seizures** <br> • **Intellectual disability** <br> • **Characteristic EEG** |
| **What is the characteristic EEG for Lennox-Gastaut patients?** | **Long runs of bilaterally synchronous sharp and slow-wave complexes – cycles at 2 per second** <br><br> *(commonly known as "atypical spike & wave pattern")* |
| What is the clinical presentation of a child with Lennox-Gastaut syndrome? | A mix of tonic, atonic, absence seizures, and tonic-clonic seizures – *most children have two or more different seizure types each day* |
| What is the drug of choice for Lennox-Gastaut syndrome? | There isn't one – it is refractory to treatment |
| Older children with Lennox-Gastaut are more likely to have which seizure type? | Tonic-clonic |
| Will children outgrow Lennox-Gastaut? | No |
| **With closed head trauma, what major risk factors make the child more likely to have a lasting seizure disorder?** | **Structural damage (cerebral contusion, hematoma, & penetrating head injury) or unconsciousness lasting >24 h** |
| **If a child or adolescent suffers a closed head trauma, loses consciousness for a few moments, then seizes, do you need to worry about ongoing seizure disorder?** | Not clear – *Note: This is a change!* <br><br> **It was previous thought that most post-traumatic seizures are benign. Recent evidence is mixed, though. Early seizures following closed head trauma *may increase risk* for ongoing seizure disorder.** |

Children who have a posttraumatic seizure are at increased risk for what seizure complication, compared to adults?

Status epilepticus is much more common in young children, with posttraumatic seizure

If a first seizure occurs within 1 week of a closed head trauma, what is the name for that seizure?

Early posttraumatic

If a seizure happens months to years after a closed head trauma, what is the name for that seizure?

Late posttraumatic

In a tonic-clonic seizure, which happens first, the tonic movement or the clonic movement?

Tonic – that's why it comes first in the name!

What other changes typically accompany a tonic-clonic seizure, in addition to the characteristics movements?

Salivation, diaphoresis, increased BP, *dilated pupils*

What is it called when the EEG shows seizure activity, but the patient's only symptom is loss of some language skills?

Acquired Epileptic Aphasia (aka Landau-Kleffner syndrome)

What is the course of acquired epileptic aphasia?

3/4 of kids will have long-term language deficits

Do antiseizure meds help with acquired epileptic aphasia?

No

(seizures may be controlled, but the language disability remains)

A complex partial seizure with the main symptom being sudden in appropriate laughter is also known as a _____?

Gelastic seizure (usually due to hypothalamic tumors)

What is cursive epilepsy?

Complex partial seizure with running as the main symptom

What is reflex epilepsy?

Seizures triggered by a particular stimulus (e.g., a certain visual pattern or touch)

**What is epilepsia partialis continua?**

Status epilepticus *with a focal seizure only (aka partial seizure)*

**It is what it sounds like**
**Epilepsia = epilepsy**
**Partialis = partial seizure**
**Continua = continuous**

**Epilepsia partialis continua usually occurs in what age group?**

<10 years

**What is Rasmussen syndrome?**

**A subacute inflammatory encephalitis associated with epilepsia partialis continua**

(probably follows an infection such as CMV – it may be due to autoantibodies activating glutamate receptors)

What is the prognosis for children with Rasmussen syndrome?

Usually stabilizes – produces hemiplegia, hemianopsia, and intellectual disability/ aphasia (depending on location of seizure activity)

Occasionally lethal

How is Rasmussen syndrome treated?

Antiseizure meds have variable effect – Surgical excision of focus often helpful (including hemispherectomy, in some cases)

Although status epilepticus requires seizure activity without full recovery for 30 minutes, when should you begin treating the patient for status epilepticus? (please note that some texts use 20 minutes)

If seizure activity lasts 10 minutes – the vast majority of seizures are only 1–2 minutes long, so if it goes 10 minutes you need to take action before permanent damage develops

**Why is valproate usually avoided in young children?**

**Higher risk of hepatotoxicity**

**Which antibiotic must you avoid in kids taking carbamazepine?**

**Erythromycin**

**Carbamazepine is mainly used for which type(s) of seizures?**

**Partial seizures**
**(any type)**

| | |
|---|---|
| **For generalized tonic-clonic seizures, which antiseizure meds are used most in children? (3)** | **Valproate & carbamazepine** **Levetiracetam use is increasing (good side effect profile)** |
| **For complex partial seizures, which antiseizure meds are most commonly used?** | **Carbamazepine & oxcarbazepine** **Phenytoin & valproate also acceptable** |
| **Ethosuximide is the drug of choice for which type of seizure?** | **Absence** |
| **When a patient has trouble with multiple seizure types, the only antiseizure med likely to help is _____?** | **Valproate** |
| **Phenobarbital is a fairly common antiseizure med in young children. Why should it be avoided in older patients?** | **Cognition and behavior significantly impaired with long-term use** |
| Which patient group does better with status epilepticus – adults or kids? | Kids |
| **What is most important to preserving the neurological function of a patient in status epilepticus?** | **ABCs – the damage mainly comes from hypoxia, hypotension, and hyperthermia** |
| What IV fluid should you give to a patient in status? | Something with a little glucose (e.g., D10) – provide the brain with a little energy substrate |
| What is the progression of medications you should try for a patient in status epilepticus? | 1. Benzos 2. Fosphenytoin (rapid IV formulation) 3. Phenobarb 4. Pentobarb coma (call anesthesia to do this) |
| **Is it alright to allow a patient on seizure medication to breast feed?** | **Yes –** Phenobarb, primidone & benzodiazepines can cause sleepiness in the infant, but are still okay |

**What are the pharmacokinetics of phenytoin (what is its pattern of elimination)?**

Zero order

(eliminated at constant rate independent of concentration)

What is the most common reason for a seizure occurring in the first 24 h after birth?

Birth hypoxia

If a full-term neonate has a single seizure due to birth hypoxia, what is the infant's most likely long-term neurological prognosis?

Normal!

A bad episode of birth hypoxia can lead to what dreaded complication?

Multisystem organ failure

Premature and "very low birth weight" infants often score no higher than six on the Apgar. Why?

Minimal tone and minimal reflex irritability (neurological system is immature)

What is the utility of a partial exchange transfusion (PET) in the treatment of polycythemia?

1. It may or may not decrease neurological sequelae
2. It increases NEC and other GI disorders

**Neural tube defects are the hallmark of what teratogenic medication's fetal syndrome?**

**Valproate**

What two organ systems are most commonly affected in fetal cocaine syndrome?

GU & CNS

An irritable, small for gestational age infant, with signs of opiate withdrawal is likely suffering from what syndrome?

Fetal cocaine syndrome

**What physical finding may be present in an infant with hydrocephalus that would not be seen in an older child?**

**Increased head circumference**

When can cerebral ventricular dilation be a normal finding?

Ventricular dilation often precedes head growth in normal infants

| | |
|---|---|
| **What is "communicating hydrocephalus?"** | **The CSF passes normally through the ventricles and base of the brain (but is blocked elsewhere)** |
| What is hydrocephalus ex vacuo? | Ventricular dilation based on loss of cerebral tissue |
| What is the most common cause of hydrocephalus ex vacuo in infants? | Periventricular leukomalacia/ periventricular hemorrhage with infarct |
| **Obstruction in the CSF system between the third ventricle and cisterna magna is what type of hydrocephalus?** | **Noncommunicating** |
| **How is macrocephaly defined?** | **Head circumference ≥2 standard deviations above average** (>95th percentile) |
| **What is the significance of macrocephaly without hydrocephalus?** | **Usually none (familial)** **(occasionally related to metabolic or neurocutaneous diseases)** |
| Is excessive production of CSF a cause of hydrocephalus? | Rarely (occasionally seen with choroid plexus tumors) |
| **Congenital aqueductal stenosis is responsible for what proportion of neonatal hydrocephalus?** | **1/3** |
| **Congenital aqueductal stenosis is an inherited disorder. How is it inherited?** | **X-linked recessive (occasionally autosomal recessive)** |
| What percentage of infants with hydrocephalus have a breech presentation? | 30 % |
| **What percentage of infants with neural tube defects develop hydrocephalus?** | **Most (90 %)** |

If an infant has an intraventricular hemorrhage, what proportion of these infants develop hydrocephalus?

**About 1/4**
**(3/4 resolve or stop expanding on their own)**

What three possible courses might an infant with posthemorrhagic hydrocephalus follow?

1. **Spontaneous resolution or no more expansion (40 %)**
2. **Persistent dilation (50 %)**
3. **Rapid dilation (10 %)**

If possible, the course of hydrocephalus is usually observed over what time period?

**Four weeks**

How reliable is papilledema as a sign of increased ICP/ hydrocephalus in a neonate?

Not reliable

What are some typical signs of hydrocephalus developing in a neonate?
(4 findings on head exam)

1. Tense fontanelle
2. Wide skull sutures
3. Prominent scalp veins
4. Rapidly increasing head circumference

Vomiting, lethargy, or irritability, apnea & bradycardia are typical general signs seen in infants with what common mechanical CNS problem?

Hydrocephalus

What is "setting sun sign," as related to hydrocephalus?

**Sclerae visible above the irises (associated with developing hydrocephalus in infants)**

At what week of pregnancy can in utero hydrocephaly often be diagnosed?

About week 16
(LMP)

How quickly will head circumference increase if rapidly expanding hydrocephalus is developing?

**>2 cm per week**

**If a neonate is developing hydrocephalus, why should you pay special attention to the thumb exam?**

**Flexion thumb deformity – 50 % of aqueductal stenosis patients have it**

You have just examined an apparently healthy, but macrocephalic infant. You have checked the parietal head circumference, and it is large. What else should you do?

Nothing – unless the child develops signs of increasing ICP

**A "cerebral bruit" suggests what cause of hydrocephalus?**

**AVM of the great vein of Galen (innominate vein enlarges in chest with this)**

How sensitive is a cranial ultrasound for detection of hydrocephalus?

98 % at 2 weeks after birth

**How often should ultrasounds for following hydrocephalus be <u>routinely</u> repeated?**

**Every 1–2 weeks**

**If a cranial ultrasound suggests hydrocephalus, but clinical exam is negative for signs of elevated ICP, what should you do?**

**Serial ultrasounds – + ultrasound findings often precede clinical findings (sometimes by a few weeks)**

**Cranial ultrasound should be used routinely to screen infants less than what birth weight?**

**1,500 g**

**If hydrocephalus is detected in utero, what is the initial management of choice?**

**C-section delivery – if the lungs are mature**

If the fetal lungs are not mature, what are the management options for hydrocephalus detected in utero?

1. Give steroids and deliver ASAP
2. Place shunt in utero

What medication can be useful to decrease CSF production in hydrocephalic infants?

Acetazolamide

| | |
|---|---|
| Hydrocephalus resulting from mechanical obstruction requires what type of treatment? | Shunting (VP or other ventricular shunt type) |
| What temporary mechanical measure can be used to decrease CSF pressure in communicating hydrocephalus? | Serial LP's |
| **What is the main objection to use of serial LPs in the treatment of communicating hydrocephalus?** | **1 % risk of meningitis with each puncture** |
| **What is the best permanent management for most types of hydrocephalus?** | **V-P shunting (ventriculoperitoneal shunting)** |
| In general, are neurological complications decreased by early or late (V-P) shunting? | Early |
| What age group has the highest risk of V-P shunt infection? | <6 months |
| What abdominal complications occur with V-P shunts? | 1. Organ perforation 2. Infection/abscess/peritonitis 3. Worsening of hydrocele 4. Worsening of inguinal hernia |
| **What is the typical organism and time course for V-P shunt infection?** | • **First 30 days after surgery** • **Staph epidermidis (from the surgery)** |
| What is the prognosis for hydrocephalic infants? | Good – 90 % survival & most have normal or near normal cognition |
| IVH occurring in the first 72 h of life is defined as _____? (what term?) | Early IVH (intraventricular hemorrhage) |
| During what postnatal period is IVH most common? | First 24 h (50 % of incidences) |
| **IVHs usually originate from what anatomical location?** | **The subependymal "germinal matrix"** |

| | |
|---|---|
| When does the germinal matrix "involute," or disappear? | 34 weeks after conception (36 weeks LMP) |
| Why are premature infants at such increased risk for IVH? (2 reasons) | 1. The germinal matrix vessels rupture easily<br>2. The preemie does not regulate blood pressure to the brain (high & low pressure are directly transmitted) |
| What is the term for the special cerebral blood flow regulation system in preemies? | "Pressure-passive" cerebral circulation |
| Why are preemies at special risk of IVH based on elevated cerebral venous pressures? | The germinal matrix is open to the cerebral venous system |
| Why do periventricular hemorrhages sometimes result in periventricular infarction? | The associated blood clot may cause enough "back pressure" to produce arterial ischemia and infarct |
| Is periventricular leukomalacia the same as periventricular hemorrhagic infarct? | No – PVL is *not caused* by IVH & is bilaterally symmetric (infarcts are caused by IVH & are unilateral) |
| Why is it a bad idea to damage your germinal matrix? | This matrix produces the neurons & glia. Its loss may affect cortical organization, growth, and myelinization |
| **What are the main risk factors for IVH?** | 1. **Severe prematurity**<br>2. **Anything that elevates BP (labor, seizures, abdominal exam, vigorous resuscitation)**<br>3. **Anything that lowers O$_2$** |
| **What is the preferred diagnostic for IVH? What are good alternatives?** | • **Ultrasound** (preferred)<br>• **CT or MRI** |
| **What is the best technique for US scanning of IVH?** | **Posterior fontanelle** |
| **When should infants <1,500 g receive IVH screening?** | **Ultrasound screening is indicated even if the infant is asymptomatic** |

| | |
|---|---|
| Shortly after an IVH, LP results will frequently "look like" the consequence of what procedural problem? | Traumatic tap |
| What percentage of LPs are negative in infants with confirmed IVH? | 20 % |
| Persistent changes in CSF following an IVH often mimic what other important disorder? | Meningitis (elevated protein & WBCs, decreased glucose) |
| LPs from neonates with IVH frequently mimic what other three situations/conditions? | 1. Normal<br>2. Traumatic tap<br>3. Meningitis |
| Elevation of what blood test suggests severe IVH has happened (or is about to happen)? | Nucleated erythrocytes |
| What is the relationship between indomethacin and IVH, when it is used as a tocolytic agent? | It <u>increases</u> IVH (and many other bad disorders) |
| What is the relationship between postnatal indomethacin and IVH? | IV indomethacin seems to decrease both incidence and severity of IVH<br><br>(low dose given in the first 3 days of life or so)<br><br>*(long-term neurodevelopmental benefit unclear, though – a separate mechanism may be involved in the neurodevelopmental outcome)* |
| How can indomethacin be used as a tocolytic, given its impact on the ductus arteriosus (closes it)? | NSAIDs such as indomethacin only close the ductus for infants in the third trimester. Indomethacin is therefore sometimes used for preterm labor in the second trimester |
| Are antenatal steroids useful for IVH prevention? | Yes (independent of effect on lung maturity) |
| Is vitamin K useful in prevention of IVH? | No (although it should be given in any case) |

In addition to tocolysis, what other positive effect may magnesium sulfate have on VLBW infants, when it is used before birth?

Reduced CP (cerebral palsy)

(it may also reduce incidence of IVH, but not as dramatically as steroid administration)

Acutely, what are the two guiding principles in managing IVH?

1. Supportive care
2. Avoid arterial or venous pressure variation

How might UACs (umbilical artery catheters) contribute to IVH?

They produce changes in cerebral blood flow velocities when samples are taken from the catheter

In addition to indomethacin and ibuprofen, what two other medications may be helpful in preventing IVH (after birth)?

1. Vitamin E (increases risk of sepsis, however)
2. Vecuronium
(paralysis in the first few days of life reduces venous/arterial BP variation – no clear data on how useful chemical paralysis is, though)

**What complications would you worry about in an infant receiving Mg sulfate?**

1. **Apnea**
2. **Hypotension (at higher concentrations)**
3. **Also slows the gut, but not an acute problem**

**How is cerebral perfusion pressure (the main determinant of cerebral blood flow) calculated?**

**$MAP - ICP = CPP$**
**Mean arterial pressure – Intracranial pressure = Cerebral perfusion pressure**

What is the most common cause of neonatal seizures?

Perinatal asphyxia

How is the type of seizure typically seen in premature neonates suffering from perinatal asphyxia different from the type seen in full-term neonates?

Full term:
    Multifocal clonic
Preemie:
    Generalized tonic

(Tonic comes first in "tonic-clonic," so that's how you can remember that younger babies/preemies tend to have tonic, while full term tend to have clonic)

In addition to perinatal asphyxia, what are three other common causes of neonatal seizures?

1. Intracranial hemorrhage (various types)
2. Metabolic derangements
3. Infection

**What type of seizure usually occurs in a neonate with a subdural hemorrhage?**

**Focal
(the irritation is in a specific brain location)**

What are the three metabolic causes of neonatal seizures you should investigate in any seizing infant?

1. *Hypoglycemia*
2. Hypocalcemia (also check magnesium)
3. Hypo/hypernatremia

What are the usual causes of hyponatremia in a neonate?
(2)

1. Iatrogenic
   (poor fluid management)
2. SIADH

What other important electrolyte needs to be checked in any hypocalcemic neonate?

Magnesium
(as with potassium, if magnesium is not adequate, calcium repletion will not work)

**What are "subtle seizures?"**

**Those that have clear EEG findings, but are not tonic, clonic, or myoclonic**

(seen in preemies & neonates – CNS immaturity prevents "synchronous & symmetrical" seizure activity)

What are typical presentations of subtle seizures?
(4)

1. Eye deviation or blinking
2. Lipsucking/smacking/drooling
3. Routinized movements (e.g., swimming or pedaling mvmt)
4. Apnea

**What patients are most likely to have subtle seizures?**

**Preemies**

How is "convulsive apnea" different from regular (nonconvulsive) apnea?

1. Regular apnea → bradycardia
   (convulsive does not)
2. Regular apnea does not have EEG changes

**What other type of seizure is more common in premature infants?**

**Tonic seizures**

| | |
|---|---|
| Can tonic seizures be focal? | Yes |
| What types of neonatal seizures often do not have EEG evidence of seizure? | 1. Generalized tonic<br>2. Focal & multifocal myoclonic |
| How can you differentiate myoclonic seizure activity from a "jittery" baby? | Jittery babies:<br>1. Stop moving if the area is passively flexed<br>2. Do not have abnormal eye movements<br>3. Move in response to a stimulus (although the stimulus is not always obvious) |
| Why is a head CT often helpful in neonates with seizures, in addition to ultrasound? | CT provides much more structural information<br>(calcifications, infarcts, malformations, etc.) |
| **What two types of amino acid diseases are causes of neonatal seizure?** | **1. Maple syrup urine disease**<br>**2. Urea cycle disorders** |
| **What ABG finding is a clue to the possible presence of urea cycle disorders?** | **Respiratory alkalosis**<br>(the respiratory center is directly stimulated by circulating ammonia, much as it is with salicylic acid) |
| When is the diagnostic value of an EEG at its peak? | The first few days after seizure onset |
| Why is rapid intervention important with seizures? | 1. To prevent hypoxia<br>(depending on seizure type)<br>2. To prevent CNS damage from *lengthy* or *repeated* seizures |
| Is lorazepam (Ativan) safe to use in neonatal seizures? | Yes |
| What are the typical first and second-line agents for control of neonatal seizures? | 1. Phenobarbital<br>2. Phenytoin |
| Where do most encephaloceles occur? | Occipital brain<br>(85 %) |

| | |
|---|---|
| What *is* an encephalocele? | Brain tissue herniated outside the cranial cavity<br>(usually covered) |
| **What is the more specific name for the most severe form of spina bifida?** | **Myelomeningocele** |
| What is a meningocele? | Only the meninges are outside the vertebral column |
| Are myelomeningoceles generally covered or uncovered? | Covered by meninges<br>(but rarely covered by skin) |
| If a posterior vertebral arch fails to ossify in the lower spine, but other tissues are intact, can this cause a problematic form of spina bifida occulta? | Yes – if the cord is tethered to a dermal sinus or fatty mass, bifid, or contains a thickened filum terminale, problems can still result due to stretching & damage to the cord |
| How does anencephaly happen? | The rostral end of the neural tube does <u>not</u> close (leaving the cerebral tissue dysfunctional or not formed) |
| When is the neural tube supposed to close? | The 29th day post-conception |
| **What are the three most common neural tube defects?** | 1. **Spina bifida occulta**<br>2. **Anencephaly**<br>3. **Myelomeningocele** |
| **What physical findings on the child's back suggest spina bifida occulta?**<br>    **(5)** | 1. **Skin dimples**<br>2. **Very small skin defects**<br>3. **Hair tufts**<br>4. **Lipomas**<br>5. **Hemangiomas** |
| **Which ethnic group is currently at greatest risk for neural tube defects, in the US?** | **Hispanics** |
| What group(s) of mothers are generally at highest risk for having children with neural tube defects? | 1. Low socioeconomic status<br>2. Advanced maternal age <u>and</u> very young maternal age |

| | |
|---|---|
| Are neural tube defects more common in girls or boys? | Girls – surprisingly enough! |
| **What two antiseizure medications are linked to neural tube defects?** | **Carbamazepine (1 %)**<br><br>&<br><br>**Valproic acid (5 %)** |
| **If one parent has a history of a neural tube defect him or herself, what is the probability of having a child with neural tube defect?** | **4 % (increased, but not dramatically)** |
| **What percentage of couples with children who have neural tube defect have no family history of neural tube problems?** | **95 %** |
| **If a couple has already had one child with a neural tube defect, what is the likelihood of having a second affected child?** | **About 3 %** |
| **Folic acid supplementation is very important in preventing neural tube defects. What other deficiencies contribute to neural tube defects?** | **Zinc & B12** |
| An oversupply of this molecule, (found in *"hard" water, cured meat products*, and blighted potatoes), is also linked to neural tube defects. What is the molecule? | Nitrates |
| "Meckel-Gruber" syndrome consists of occipital encephalocele, and what associated abnormalities? (5 – there can be more, but these are the essential ones) | 1. Microcephaly<br>2. Microphthalmos<br>3. Cleft lip/palate<br>4. Polydactyly<br>5. Ambiguous genitalia |
| What specialty consultation is emergently needed for children born with encephaloceles? | Neurosurgery –<br>(often the exterior tissue is damaged and must be excised, or VP shunt is needed |

| | |
|---|---|
| As in spinal cord injury, what part of the physical exam is especially important for prognostication with myelomeningocele? | **Anal tone/anal wink** (if present – "sacral sparing" is a good prognostic) |
| **What special anaphylaxis risk has been noted in infants with neural tube defects?** | **Latex allergy** (they are much more likely to have it) |
| What are the <u>initial management</u> steps for a child born with myelomeningocele? (aside from ABC's) | 1. Neurosurgical consult 2. IV antibiotics 3. NPO 4. Moist sterile wrap of exposed tissues (ask the surgeon what s/he wants – gauze is sometimes not alright) |
| In addition to performing a physical exam, what diagnostic will you want to order for infants born with myelomeningoceles? | Head CT (for hydrocephalus or other malformations) |
| **What is the usual definitive management for myelomeningocele, and why? (2 reasons)** | • **Surgical closure ≤48 h** • **Decreases infection & prevents further loss of function** |
| **When does hydrocephalus most commonly develop for infants with myelomeningocele?** | **2–3 weeks after closure** |
| How common is it for myelomeningocele patients to have or develop hydrocephalus? | Very common – 90 % |
| **Patients with myelomeningocele are still at high risk of death in the first year of life. What system is usually the source of their problems?** | **Respiratory** (apnea, aspiration, laryngeal problems) |
| **Dysfunction of, or infection from, what organ system is a frequent cause of mortality in myelomeningocele children after age 1 year?** | **GU** (neurogenic bladder leads to reflux, urosepsis, and hydronephrosis) |

| | |
|---|---|
| **Delay in walking or anal sphincter control suggests that what congenital anomaly was missed?** | **Spina bifida occulta** |
| **Foot deformity, or recurrent meningitis, can be unusual presentations of what congenital neurological abnormality?** | **Spina bifida occulta** |
| **How might an infant with hypercalcemia present?** (4) | 1. **Seizure** <br> 2. **Polyuria** <br> 3. **Lethargy** <br> 4. **Poor feeding/weight gain** <br> (low calcium can also cause seizures) |
| **What are Mg sulfate's two main effects on the body?** | 1. **CNS depressant** <br> 2. **Decreases contractility of muscle** |
| What does a neonatal seizure look like? | Subtle – <br> Staring, lip smacking, cycling movements, etc. |
| Although most neonatal seizures are due to birth asphyxia, what must you rule out before you consider asphyxia to be the cause? | Metabolic causes |
| What are the likely neurodevelopmental consequences of neonatal seizures (due to birth asphyxia)? | Usually none |
| How are neonatal seizures treated? (if not due to metabolic causes) | Phenobarbital |
| Shortly after birth, a full-term neonate develops multisystem organ failure. What is the likely cause? | Birth asphyxia – it affects <u>all</u> organs, not just the brain |
| Which medication is given to prevent seizures in Moms with preeclampsia? | Mg sulfate |

What is the main way that neonatal polycythemia causes long-term problems? | Damage to the CNS – usually multiple, subtle problems

**Very high-pitched or shrieking cries are common in which two newborn groups?**

**1. Preemies**
**2. Neurologically impaired**

**What is aplasia cutis?**

**A little bit of missing skin**

**Midline aplasia cutis suggests what problem?**

**Spinal dysraphism**
**(or cerebral problems, if it occurs on the midline scalp)**

**Multiple areas (on the scalp) of aplasia cutis indicate what disorder, classically?**

**Trisomy 13**

**A persistent posterior fontanelle + jaundice in a neonate = what disorder?**

**Hypothyroidism**

**What is Harlequin skin?**

**A baby that is half pink and half pale, divided down the midline**

**What is the pathological significance of Harlequin skin?**

**None**

(It sometimes occurs in young babies laid on their side, due to immaturity of the cutaneous vessel tone mechanism)

**What is the earliest sign of craniosynostosis?**

**Increasing bone density at the suture line**

**Are neurological complications common if craniosynostosis is isolated (single suture)?**

**No**

If multiple sutures are involved in craniosynostosis, what general concept should you think of? | Congenital syndromes

**In a neonate, Horner's syndrome is often due to _____?**

**Lower brachial plexus injury**

| | |
|---|---|
| How does Horner's syndrome present in neonates? | **Ptosis, miosis,** & *enophthalmos (sunken eye)*<br><br>*(impaired facial flushing can also occur, giving a "harlequin" appearance on the face)* |
| When neurologically evaluating a newborn, should flexion or extension be greater? | **Always flexion** |
| Do normal term infants have normal deep tendon reflexes? | **Yes** |
| What is the "finger grasp" reflex? | **Putting something into the baby's palm makes him/her flex & hold on** |
| What does the baby do in the "Moro" reflex? | **Throws its arms out with palms open** |
| Migratory clonic seizures in the first 24 h of life are characteristic of what type of birth problem? | **Asphyxia** |
| What unusual pupillary finding is seen with asphyxia injuries in the first 24 h? | **Either constriction or dilation**<br><br>**(constriction is worse)** |
| What are the most common anomalies seen in infants of diabetic mothers? | 1. **VSD**<br>2. **Neural tube defects**<br>3. **GI atresia**<br>4. **Urinary tract malformations** |
| In "acute kernicterus," how many symptom phases do you see? | **Three** |
| Phase I kernicterus has what type of symptoms? | **Low stuff mainly –**<br>**Low tone (hypotonia)**<br>**Low suck**<br>**Low level of consciousness (stupor)**<br>**Seizures (low neural inhibition)** |

| | |
|---|---|
| The middle phase of kernicterus features what symptoms? | Mainly overactivity/high stuff<br>1. Hypertonia (extensors)<br>2. Opisthotonous (posture)<br>3. Retrocollis<br>4. Fever<br><br>(retrocollis is backward Arching of the neck not due to meningitic irritation) |
| The final phase of acute kernicterus is simply hypertonia. What happens in the chronic phase? | A mix of high & low stuff<br>Low – hypotonia & delayed motor skills<br><br>High – DTRs & tonic neck reflexes |
| If a baby with a history of high bilirubin is now hypertonic, but doesn't have fever or any funny posturing, what does the infant have? | Phase 3 of acute kernicterus |
| The ash leaf spots of tuberous sclerosis can be identified on physical exam with what special technique? | They fluoresce with a Woods lamp |
| How does tick paralysis look different from Guillain-Barré? | The paralysis develops in just hours with tick paralysis – G-B usually takes days |
| Why are reflexes missing in Guillain-Barré? | Lower motor neurons are not functioning |
| How is Guillain-Barré treated? | IVIG & Plasmapheresis<br><br>(steroids and immunosuppressives are sometimes also used) |
| What is the natural course of Guillain-Barré? | Slow improvement, as long as respiration and autonomic function is supported |
| A vignette that describes an adolescent with jerky movements while trying to eat his breakfast cereal, or dropping soap in the shower quite often, is probably describing which disorder? | Juvenile myoclonic epilepsy |

**What happens if a myasthenia gravis patient is given succinylcholine or another paralytic agent?**

**Paralysis can last for days or weeks!**

**Transverse myelitis is typically triggered by what two events?**

**A viral infection (or flu-like illness)**

**OR**

**Vaccination**

(always consider multiple sclerosis when transverse myelitis is diagnosed – it is a fairly common first MS presentation, and changes management after the acute phase)

**What is the most commonly identified cause of transverse myelitis in children, or is it most commonly idiopathic?**

**Idiopathic**

(estimates vary depending which literature you read, but has been quoted as 89 % idiopathic in pediatric literature)

**Is transverse myelitis an upper motor neuron problem, or lower?**

**Upper – at least one horizontal segment of the cord is affected**

**("extensive" pediatric transverse myelitis affects at least 3 levels, and often as much as 6!)**

**How does transverse myelitis usually present?**

**Abrupt onset of:**
**1. Back pain that radiates to front**
**2. Lower extremity weakness**
**3. Frequent loss of bladder control**
**(may also include autonomic instability)**

**What is the usual course of transverse myelitis?**

**Spontaneous resolution over weeks, About 40 % have full return of function**

**Remainder have residual deficits of varying severity**

**How is acute transverse myelitis in children usually treated, if no underlying cause can be found?**

**High-dose steroids for 5–7 days (reduces length of disability & improves outcomes)**

**Then**

**Slow oral steroid taper (over weeks)**

| | |
|---|---|
| Are motor or sensory fibers affected in transverse myelitis? | Both – at and below the affected part of the cord |
| How is transverse myelitis differentiated clinically from other related disorders producing weakness (e.g., ischemic or hereditary myelopathy)? | The nadir of function generally occurs between 4 h and 21 days following symptom onset |
| If a neonate has a seizure, should an LP be performed? | Unless there is a mass lesion, yes. |
| Which electrolyte abnormalities are most likely to result in neonatal seizures? | Hypoglycemia & hypocalcemia |
| If an infant has seizures in the neonatal period, and anti-seizure medications are needed, when is it appropriate to stop those medications? | One month after the last seizure (if the neuro exam is normal) |
| If a child has a history of seizure without a fever, then later has a seizure while febrile, could the second seizure be considered a "febrile seizure?" | No – criteria require that the patient has no seizure history other than prior febrile seizures |
| What is a "simple" febrile seizure? (3 criteria) | 1. Lasts less than 15 min 2. Non-focal 3. No more than one per febrile illness |
| What is the typical age for febrile seizures? | 6 months to 6 years (some sources state 3 months to 5 years, but 6 & 6 is frequently quoted & easy to remember) |
| Most febrile seizures occur in what smaller age range? | 14–22 months The peak incidence is at about 18 months |
| Administration of which vaccine has been associated with a doubling in the febrile seizure rate? | MMR or MMRV (with varicella) *IF first dose given after 15 months!* |

| | |
|---|---|
| Is the rate of rise in temperature the most important determinant of whether a febrile seizure will happen for children predisposed to have a febrile seizure? | **No –** **It is clear that fever must be present. Exactly what about the fever makes the febrile seizure likely is not clear.** *This is a change – recent data do not support the "rate of rise" hypothesis* |
| Which infections are especially associated with febrile seizures? | **Roseola (HHV-6)** **Shigella** |
| What are the main patient characteristics that increase risk for febrile seizures? (4) | 1. **Family history (!!!)** 2. **Daycare attendance** 3. **Developmental delay** 4. **Required >28 days treatment in a neonatal unit** |
| Should EEG be used in the evaluation of febrile seizure? | **No** |
| Do febrile seizures damage the brain? | **No** |
| Should children with febrile seizures be put on antiseizure medication? | **No** |
| What treatment is approved for children who have frequent febrile seizures? | **Oral or rectal diazepam (valium) to be given when fever is noticed** **(Cost/benefit should be weight, though!)** |
| What proportion of children who have a febrile seizure will never have another seizure? | 2/3 (IF the child has a second febrile seizure, it is usually within 1 year of the first one) |
| If a child has two febrile seizures, what is the probability that he/she will have more? | **About ½** |

**Which kids are at greatest risk for recurrent febrile seizures? (4 factors)**

The ones who were most easily provoked into having a seizure:

1. **Seizure happened with a low-grade temp**
2. **Seizure happened shortly after the temp began**
3. **Seizure happened in one of the kid's first febrile experiences (<18 months old)**

**+ those with a first-degree relative who had febrile seizures**

**Do children who have a febrile seizure have an increased risk of later epilepsy?**

**Yes, but it is still very low**
(It was traditionally reported as double the risk, but some data shows it could be as much as five times higher. However, the general population's epilepsy risk is approximately 0.5, so quite low)

Is aura before a migraine common in children?

No – fairly common in adults, but not in kids

**What special type of migraine typically presents in adolescent girls with vertigo, syncope, and dysarthria?**

**Basilar artery migraine**

Which migraine is associated with a patient who becomes deeply confused, and stays that way for hours?

Confusional migraine

(Finally, a name that makes sense!)

Weakness on one side of the body, sometimes accompanied by aphasia, which resolves and then recurs (but does *not* change sides) could be what type of migraine?

Hemiplegic (the paralysis can last for days)

**What are the characteristics of a migraine headache? (4)**

**Pain on one side**
**Pulsatile or throbbing pain**
**Moderate to severe, & worse with activity**
**+/– nausea, photophobia, phonophobia**

| | |
|---|---|
| How is migraine treated in children? | First line – acetaminophen or ibuprofen<br>Second line – triptans (e.g., sumatriptan) |
| What is the main medication used to prevent migraine headaches in children? | Propranolol |
| **How long must a headache last to possibly qualify as a migraine?** | 4–72 h |
| **How many times must a person have a headache that qualifies as a migraine, to be considered to have migraines?** | 5 |
| **If a child complains of a headache, then has a seizure, does that warrant getting a head CT?** | Yes |
| **If a headache wakes a child from sleep, or is present when he/she wakes up, is it reasonable to scan the head?** | Yes |
| **A child has two febrile seizures in 6 months. Should he be started on antiseizure medication?** | No |
| **What is the other "no-brainer" for when to order a head CT for a headache patient?** | **Abnormal or focal neuro exam** |
| **What is the underlying problem for myasthenia gravis patients?** | **Antibodies to the ACh receptor**<br><br>**(the antibodies cause two problems:**<br>**1. They block the receptors**<br>**2. They cause the receptors to be eaten up by the immune system)** |
| **What is "juvenile" myasthenia gravis?** | **Myasthenia gravis that develops in childhood – usually in kids ≥10 years old** |
| **How does juvenile myasthenia gravis present?** | **Same as in adults – ocular muscle problems, ptosis, dysarthria, and muscles that fatigue with increased use** |

**Which medication is used to test for myasthenia gravis (MG)?**

**Edrophonium aka the Tensilon test**

**What *kind* of medication is used to test for myasthenia?**

**Acetylcholinesterase inhibitor**

**(increases the concentration of ACh, transiently improving muscle function via the receptors still present)**

How is myasthenia gravis treated (juvenile or adult form)?

Oral anticholinesterase meds
Immunosuppressants
Plasmapheresis (mainly short-term use)
IVIG (better tolerated than plasmapheresis)
Thymectomy

What is the main use for IVIG therapy in myasthenia patients?

Treatment of MG crisis, or those with severe weakness not responding to other treatments

**Why is Guillain-Barré syndrome dangerous?**

**Two reasons –**
**Respiratory muscles can be paralyzed &
Autonomic instability can develop**

**How does Guillain-Barré present?**

**Ascending weakness – usually following a viral illness**

**Does Guillain-Barré affect motor fibers, sensory fibers, or both?**

**Motor**

Which bacterial infections are especially associated with the later development of Guillain-Barré?

Campylobacter & Mycoplasma

**How is a lumbar puncture helpful in diagnosing Guillain-Barré?**

**Few WBCs, but *high protein***

Which medications should you avoid when treating Guillain-Barré patients, due to a possibly life-threatening complication?

Antihypertensives

(At risk for severe hypotension)

How is Guillain-Barré treated?

Supportive care –
Plasmapheresis and IVIG may shorten recovery time

| | |
|---|---|
| What is the typical course for Guillain-Barré? | Full recovery within 6 months (usually takes just 3–4 weeks) |
| **An infant presents with poor feeding, hypotonia, constipation, ptosis, facial weakness, and dry mouth. Diagnosis?** | **Infantile botulism**<br><br>**(dry mouth/absence of secretions helps you to differentiate it from other low tone states)** |
| **How is infantile botulism definitively diagnosed?** | **Stool samples showing *C. botulinum* or the toxin** |
| **How do older children with botulism present differently from infants?** | **Blurry vision, double vision, nausea & vomiting are more prominent – still have overall weakness, most noticeable initially in the cranial nerves** |
| **For older children with botulism poisoning, what therapy can be given?** | **Antitoxin**<br><br>**(there is a new *heptavalent* antitoxin recommended for patients ≥1 year old – it treats all known types of botulinum toxin)** |
| **If you botulism patient is <1 year old, is there a way to treat him or her?** | **Yes –**<br>**Human-derived immunoglobulin (viral screen & detergent washed)**<br><br>***Known as "BabyBIG"***<br>***(Baby Botulinum ImmunoGlobulin)*** |
| **What is the limitation to treatment with BabyBIG?** | **It treats only botulinum neurotoxins A & B (the most common ones for infants, but not the only possible ones)** |
| Do antibiotics help in treating botulism? | If the source is a wound, then yes (penicillin may be used)<br><br>If the toxin was ingested, then no |
| **In what part of the skull do most skull fractures occur?** | **The parietal lobe** |

| | |
|---|---|
| **What physical findings suggest basilar skull fractures?** | 1. **Raccoon eyes**<br>2. **Battle's sign (ecchymosis over the mastoid area)**<br>3. **Otorrhea (of CSF)**<br>4. **Rhinorrhea (of CSF)**<br>5. **Hemotympanum (blood behind the TM)** |
| Air inside the head suggests that what type of injury has happened? | Fracture of a sinus<br>(that connects to the intracerebral space) |
| **What management is needed for a non-depressed linear skull fracture?** | **None – follow-up X-ray should be done in 3–6 months to show that it is healing properly** |
| **In children <3 years old, skull X-rays can be done after head trauma. When would a head CT be a better choice?** | **Any time you want information about the underlying tissue –**<br><br>Focal neuro examination<br>Abnormal neuro exam<br>Very young child (<6 months)<br>Loss of consciousness >5 min<br>Seizures |
| If a patient has CSF otorrhea or rhinorrhea, what should s/he avoid doing (which is tough)? | Sneezing or coughing |
| **Which sort of skull fracture definitely requires inpatient observation?** | **Basilar skull fracture with otorrhea or rhinorrhea** |
| **Acceleration-deceleration mechanism of injury is most associated with what CNS problem?** | **Diffuse axonal shear injury**<br><br>(shearing at the white/gray matter junction) |
| Is a scalp laceration dangerous? | Yes – they bleed like crazy, and can cause *exsanguination!* |
| Are scalp hematomas dangerous in toddlers and older children? | No |
| **What is an epidural hematoma?** | **Blood collecting between the skull and the dura mater** |

| | |
|---|---|
| **What causes an epidural hematoma?** | **Tear of the middle meningeal artery (which runs along the temporal bone) is nearly always the reason** |
| **What is the typical vignette for an epidural hematoma?** | **Someone is hit with a bat on the temple. Initially he/she passes out, then regains consciousness and is basically fine, then rapidly goes downhill and dies** |
| **Classically, how should an epidural hematoma look on head CT?** | **White and lens shaped** |
| **Which type of hematoma can cross the suture lines of the skull – subdural or epidural?** | **Subdural – there is nothing much between it and the brain, so the spread of fluid is not affected by suture lines at all** |
| **Which one is more likely to cause a seizure, subdural or epidural hematoma?** | **Subdural**<br><br>**(the blood against the brain irritates the neurons, leading to seizure activity)** |
| Which one typically expands faster, epidural or subdural hematoma? | Epidural – it is usually due to arterial bleeding, so it expands quickly |
| What kind of bleeding usually produces a subdural hematoma? | Venous |
| **Following head trauma, a child develops bradycardia, hypertension, and elevated ICP. Why?** | **Elevated ICP causes reflex bradycardia, hypertension, and changes in respiratory pattern –**<br><br>**It is called "Cushing's triad"** (generated by Cushing's reflex of ↑ICP causing changes in sympathetic & parasympathetic outflow) |
| Which is more likely to produce herniation, epidural or subdural? | Epidural – because the change in pressure is faster |
| **What are the early signs of herniation with epidural hematoma?**<br>  (3 main physical exam signs) | • **3rd nerve palsy**<br>• **"Blown" pupil on side of lesion**<br>• **Progressive hemiplegia same side as lesion** |

**In what situation are chronic subdural hematomas most commonly seen in children (subdurals present for more than 3 weeks)?**

**Shaken-baby syndrome**

**(although some subdurals are due to other types of head trauma, intentional & unintentional)**

**What is the most common cause of spinal cord injury in infants?**

**Birth trauma**
(due to torsion or traction forces)

**What are the three common mechanisms of spinal cord injury in children?**

1. **Motor vehicle collisions**
2. **Falls**
3. **Diving injury**

Children <3 years old have an increased chance of injuring what part(s) of the spine?

Cervical and thoracic

What is the Gallant response?

A reflex that allows you to check thoracic spinal function *in newborns*

(scratching in the thoracic paraspinal area makes them curve the spine toward the scratch if the cord is intact)

If the spinal cord, or a higher motor area, is injured, what is the initial response by the involved muscles?

They are flaccid

What happens over the first few weeks following an upper motor neuron lesion (spinal cord or brain)?

The involved muscles become spastic/ hyperreflexic

Following spinal cord injury, what treatment should you provide?

High-dose methylprednisolone

**A patient comes in to the ER who seems to have a C-spine fracture, but has also dislocated his shoulder. The shoulder needs to go back in or it may suffer permanent damage. Can you manipulate the patient to get it back in?**

**No – C-spine takes priority and you cannot guarantee that it won't move during the reduction/relocation**

| | |
|---|---|
| When the sciatic nerve is injured in kids, what is the usual reason? | IM injection of the buttocks (that's why we don't use that location in young kids) |
| In infants, what is the most common cause of peripheral nerve injury? | Birth trauma |
| Which peripheral nerve injury is *most common* for infants? | Upper brachial plexus injury (Erb-Duchenne palsy – the one with the droopy shoulder and inwardly rotated arm, with the hand ready to get a "tip") |
| How likely is it that a child with an upper plexus injury will recover fully? | Very likely – 90 % without surgery |
| What is the eponymic name for lower brachial plexus nerve injury? | Klumpke-Dejerine palsy/injury |
| What does a lower plexus injury look like on physical exam? | The hand and forearm are paralyzed, with sensory and vasomotor abnormalities |
| Which has a better prognosis, upper brachial plexus injury in infancy, or lower brachial plexus injury in infancy? | Upper (although the majority of lower lesions will also spontaneously improve) |
| What is the second most common *lethal* autosomal recessive disorder? | Spinal muscle atrophy (SMA) (the worst form of which is Werdnig-Hoffman) |
| What is the guiding principle in understanding the prognosis for a patient with a particular SMA? | The earlier the onset, the worse the prognosis (& the more rapid the progression) |
| What is the buzzword for Werdnig-Hoffman? | Tongue fasciculations! |
| Why do Werdnig-Hoffman patients die? | Respiratory muscle weakness (usually dead by 2 years old) |

**How do Werdnig-Hoffman patients present?**

Weakness & hypotonia by 6 months old

What is special about the presentation of spinal muscle atrophy type II?

- Initially normal milestones, but then have difficulty with independent sitting & do not stand
- Weakness plateaus, then worsens when an intercurrent illness occurs

(most die by age 20 & often earlier, mainly due to complications of respiratory infection)

What is the fate of Kugelberg-Welder SMA (type III)?

They survive, can stand & walk

Trouble with further motor tasks, such as stair climbing

(Bulbar dysfunction develops late in the course)

Overall normal life expectancy

At what age does Kugelberg-Welder SMA (type III) present?

After 18 months

What causes spinal muscle atrophy disorders?

Degeneration of the anterior horn cells (as in polio)

What critical planning issue needs to be addressed with the families of SMA patients, who have more rapidly progressive forms?

Tracheostomy/long-term ventilatory support (before respiratory arrest occurs!)

(In general, long-term care goals balancing life-extending interventions with comfort & palliative care need to be set)

Do kids with SMA have high or normal CPK?

Normal – the problem is in the neurons, not the muscle cells

**Do Duchenne muscular dystrophy patients have normal or high CPK?**

High

**When will boys with Duchenne muscular dystrophy lose the ability to walk?**

Around age 11

| | |
|---|---|
| **How is the diagnosis of muscular dystrophy made?** | **Biopsy or genetic testing** |
| **What muscle finding on physical exam is classic for Duchenne?** | **Calf "pseudohypertrophy"** <br> **(looks like hypertrophy, but it's not)** |
| **A 4 year old boy is presented with a change in gait – Mom says he looks like a little duck now. She also notices that he often falls, probably because he's been walking on his toes. What is his most likely disorder?** | **Duchenne muscular dystrophy** <br> (the "duck walk" is usually known as a "waddling" gait) |
| What physical exam finding precedes the loss of muscle function in Duchenne? | Scoliosis <br> (accelerates rapidly once the child is in a wheelchair) |
| What is the most common cause of death for Duchenne patients? | Respiratory failure |
| **In addition to calf pseudohypertrophy, what is the other really important buzzword for Duchenne?** | **Gower's sign – the boy "walks" up his legs with his arm to assist himself to a standing position** |
| **A neonate is presented whose physical exam is notable for a cranial bruit. The child is also having problems with CHF & hydrocephalus. What is the underlying problem?** | **Great Vein of Galen malformation** <br> (the giant intracerebral vein – the CHF is due to the extra pumping needed, given that arterial blood is going into this giant vein) |
| Does a normal EEG rule out epilepsy? | No – positive findings help to make the diagnosis, but negative doesn't mean anything |
| What are the two simplest possibilities to investigate when a child on antiseizure meds has a breakthrough seizure? | 1. Noncompliance <br> 2. Weight gain/growth has made a previously effective dose too small <br><br> Check the med level and how recently it was adjusted |

| | |
|---|---|
| How common are febrile seizures? | Common –<br>3 % of kids have had one by age 5! |
| **What proportion of kids has a second febrile seizure, if they've already had the first one?** | 1/3 |
| **Are febrile seizures more likely to recur when the child is very young at the time of first seizure, or older at time of first seizure?** | Younger |
| **What information from family history will help you estimate the probability of another febrile seizure occurring for a child who's just had one?** | + family history of febrile seizures increases the probability |
| **In communicating hydrocephalus, which ventricles will dilate?** | <u>All</u> of them –<br>the problem is <u>outside</u> the ventricular system<br>(for example, fluid can't be taken up by the arachnoid granulations to return it to the venous circulation) |
| **What is anencephaly?** | When part of the brain & cranium are missing |
| Anencephaly always involves what part of the brain? | The forebrain<br>(last area to develop, so biggest chance of being messed up) |
| There are several reasons that anencephaly is usually incompatible with life. Absence of which tissues causes the biggest problem for most of these infants? | No hypothalamus, adrenals, or pituitary |
| **The main signs/symptoms of hydrocephalus in a young child are _____?**<br>   **(3)** | **Nausea/vomiting/irritability** |

| | |
|---|---|
| **The main signs/symptoms of hydrocephalus in an older child or adolescent are _____?** | **Headache – especially early morning headache**<br>**+ nausea/vomiting**<br><br>**(same signs for tumors, of course)** |
| **The most cost-effective way to diagnose hydrocephalus in a young child is _____?** | **Serial head circumference measurements** |
| If intracranial pressure is increasing, which cranial nerves are likely to develop a palsy? | 3rd & 6th<br>(oculomotor & abducens –<br>eye movements & lateral gaze) |
| If hydrocephalus is diagnosed in utero, what can you do about it? | Ventriculoamniotic shunt can be placed |
| How successful is in utero shunting at preventing later motor & cognitive problems for the infant? | About 50 % |
| Most long-term shunting connects a lateral ventricle to the peritoneum. If the shunt is connected to the atrium instead, what bad complication will sometimes develop? | Pulmonary hypertension<br>(due to microemboli showers from the shunt tip) |
| If a patient has hydrocephalus, but the hydrocephalus is increasing very slowly, and there are no bad signs/symptoms, is it alright to treat the patient medically? | Yes, but surgery is ultimately better<br><br>(agents such as furosemide and acetazolamide are used for medical management) |
| What is syringomyelia? | An abnormal cavity in the spinal cord, near the center, that often causes central cord syndrome |
| How can you recognize central cord syndrome?<br>(2 physical exam<br>& 1 history aspect) | 1. Weakness in upper extremities > than lower extremities<br>2. Distal muscles more affected than proximal<br>3. Usually follows a neck hyperextension injury |

| | |
|---|---|
| What is hydromyelia? | Expansion of an otherwise normal central spinal canal – <br> Usually asymptomatic |
| Where does spina bifida usually occur? <br> (specific segments) | L5-S1 |
| **How are most cases of spina bifida treated?** | **No treatment needed** |
| **When a dermoid sinus is present over a neural tube defect, does it generally connect to the dura or cord?** | **No –** <br><br> **if they do, the patient presents with recurrent meningitis** |
| **Meningoceles usually don't require emergent surgery. In what situations is it critical to perform rapid repair?** | **1. Leaking CSF** <br> **2. Not skin covered** <br>    **(risk of meningitis)** |
| If a couple has a child born with myelomeningocele, what is the risk of the same problem occurring in later siblings? | 3–4 % <br><br> (up from 0.1 % for the general population) |
| If a couple has two children affected by myelomeningocele, does the risk to future pregnancies increased beyond the initial 3–4 % probability? | Yes – it goes to *10 %!* |
| What is the Chiari malformation? | Cerebellar tonsils, and sometimes the brainstem and more of the cerebellum are too low – as if they slid into the spinal canal |
| What is the other name for the Chiari malformation? | Arnold-Chiari malformation |
| What other problems are associated with the Chiari malformation, in addition to the displaced structures themselves? | Hydrocephalus (sometimes) & spinal cord problems |

| | |
|---|---|
| Do Arnold-Chiari patients often have errors in the development of other systems? | No<br><br>(That's why it's a "malformation," not a syndrome) |
| What percentage of children with myelomeningocele will have hydrocephalus and type II Arnold-Chiari malformation? | 80–90 % |
| **There are three types of Chiari malformation. Which is the most common symptomatic type?** | **Type 2**<br>**(medulla & cerebellar tonsils have moved downward)** |
| Which type of Chiari malformation can be *acquired*, not just congenital? | Type 1<br>(often asymptomatic – only the cerebellar tonsils are too far down, partly through the foramen magnum – NO myelomeningocele & no brain stem involvement) |
| Which type of Chiari malformation is most common overall? | Type 1 |
| **What is type 3 Chiari malformation?** | **Cerebellum & medulla partly or fully below the foramen magnum – often in an occipital encephalocele** |
| **Type 1 Chiari malformations, and occasionally very mild type 2s, are sometimes asymptomatic. What is the most appropriate way to manage these patients?** | **Observe** |
| **Type 2 Chiari malformation is often associated with _____ & _____?** | **Hydrocephalus**<br>&<br>**Myelomeningocele** |
| Types 2 & 3 Chiari malformation are almost always obvious at birth. Type 1 often presents later. What are the usual signs of type 1? | 1. Headache<br>2. **Neck pain**<br>3. Bulbar problems/cranial nerve palsies<br>4. Sleep apnea<br>5. Ataxia |

Dandy-Walker syndrome has to do with the posterior fossa, too. How is it different from Arnold-Chiari?

1. It's a syndrome – so other organ systems are often involved.
2. The 4th ventricle turns into a giant cyst
3. The cerebellum is very small & squished into the anterior portion of the cyst

**What are the main associated problems to watch out for with Dandy-Walker patients?**

**Cardiac anomalies**

   **&**

**90 % have hydrocephalus**

**(usually all ventricles are affected, but the 4th is especially large)**

**How is Becker muscular dystrophy similar to Duchenne muscular dystrophy?**

**Symptoms are similar**

**What are the crucial differences between Duchenne muscular dystrophy and Becker muscular dystrophy?**
   **(3)**

• **Starts later**
• **Progress is slower**
• **Symptoms are less severe**

**Closed head trauma that does not result in any bleeding or swelling, but still produces a temporary period of altered consciousness, is called _____?**

**A concussion**

How many "grades" are there, when you are grading a concussion?

Three

Note: There are now several classification systems for concussions. Many clinicians have moved away from using the scoring systems, due to confusion about the best way to score them, and how useful the scoring really is. It may still be utilized on the boards, or by other clinicians with whom you speak, though.

**If your patient lost consciousness due to a closed head injury, what grade of concussion are you dealing with?**

**Three**

| | |
|---|---|
| **Following a concussion, how long must your patient avoid contact sports?** | **Until ALL symptoms, including any memory or concentration difficulties have completely resolved** |
| **What additional testing is often recommended prior to a return to contact sports, after a concussion?** | **"Provocative testing" –**<br>**Have the patient do an activity that increases BP & heart rate, such as sit-ups or jogging. Check whether any symptoms recur. IF SO, NO RETURN TO SPORTS YET** |
| **In both grades 1 and 2 concussions, the patient remains conscious. How are grades 1 and 2 different?** | **Grade 2 has amnesia for the event – Grade 1 does not** |
| **What is a grade 1 concussion?** | **Transient confusion only** |
| How long must a grade 1 concussion patient sit out from contact sports? | No return to sports until symptoms completely resolve<br><br>&<br><br>Evaluated by a medical professional |
| **What are post-concussive symptoms?** | **Dizziness**<br>**Persistent headaches**<br>**Memory problems**<br>**Difficulty sleeping/concentrating**<br>**Sensitivity to light or noise**<br>**Depression, anxiety, & fatigue** |
| **How long do symptoms from a concussion (also known as "mild traumatic brain injury" or MTBI) typically last?** | **Most have headache resolution within 2–4 weeks**<br><br>**Most have recovery of neuropsychological functions within 72 h** |
| **Why is it important to avoid a second closed head injury, if a concussion has recently occurred?** | **Increases likelihood of more serious neurological sequelae from apparently minor closed head injuries** |
| **In addition to avoiding sports or other possible head injury, how should a concussion be treated?** | **Physical & cognitive rest!** |

| Which typical sports are high risk for MTBI (concussion)? | Boxing<br>Football/rugby/soccer<br>Ice hockey<br>Wrestling |
| Do concussion patients require evaluation at a medical facility? | Grades 2 & 3 do<br><br>(Grade 1 requires medical evaluation, but not necessarily at an institution) |

# Index